MW01596635

Instruct

Contemporary
Professional
Nursing

Joseph T. Catalano, RN,PhD,CCRN
Professor of Nursing
East Central University
Ada, Oklahoma

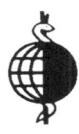

F. A. Davis Company • Philadelphia

F. A. Davis Company
1915 Arch Street
Philadelphia, PA 19103

Printed in the United States of America

ISBN 0-8036-0096-8

Chapter 1: The Development of Nursing Profession

In Chapter 1, the student is introduced to the concept of profession and how it differs from a job or occupation. The three most common approaches to defining a profession are presented with emphasis placed on the Trait *Approach*. Nursing is analyzed in relationship to the characteristics of a profession. The concept of empowerment is explored, including the nature of power and the different sources for power. The chapter concludes with a discussion of accountability and professionalism, and the need for nurses to belong to professional organizations in order to maximize their professional power.

Teaching Points

1. Identify the differences between job, occupation, and profession.
2. Present the three ways to define a profession, and how nursing measures as a profession against each approach.
3. Discuss each of the characteristics of a profession as presented in the trait approach, and compare nursing with each one. Note that nursing is still lacking in education and independence of practice.
4. Present the concept of power, why it is important in nursing, and the sources of power.
5. Identify ways that nurses can increase their power as professionals, and the power of nursing as a profession.
6. Present the concept of *accountability* as part of professionalism and why it is important.

Test Questions

1. An important element in nursing's attempt to gain full autonomy of practice includes:
   a. Economic exploitation of nurses
   b. Maintaining the education system for nurses as it is now
   c. Gaining and maintaining control of nursing practice by nurses
   d. Restricting the latitude of decisions made by nurses

2. As a general principle, whenever a person has freedom and independence, there is also:
   a. Health and happiness
   b. Chaos and disorder
   c. Loss of control and negative feedback
   d. Responsibility and accountability

3. An important method that nurses could use to gain significant power in the United States is to
   a. Use strikes and union tactics to increase pay
   b. Join professional organizations in large numbers
   c. Leave nursing as soon as better jobs came along
   d. All of the above are good ways to gain power

4. Power from close personal relationships is called:
   a. Coercive
   b. Reward
   c. Legitimate
   d. Referent

5. A group of jobs that are similar as to type of work and that are found throughout an industry or country describes:
   a. Position
   b. Occupation
   c. Profession
   d. Stint

6. Which of the following types of nurses are classified as "Technical Nurses?"
   a. BSN and MSN
   b. LPN and ADN
   c. LVN and BSN
   d. None of the above

7. "A profession is in a continual state of development on a continuum" best describes:
   a. The trait approach to professions
   b. The power approach to professions
   c. The process approach to professions
   d. The educational approach to professions

8. Which of the following would be the best indicator of increasing accountability in the profession of nursing?
   a. Increasing pay scale for staff nurses
   b. Improved public image of nurses on TV and in movies
   c. Demonstration of competency and high quality care through peer review
   d. Taking care of larger number of clients with the help of unlicensed assistive personnel

9. Which of the following would be the best method for nurses to prepare for future professional practice?
   a. Take additional courses in the use of computers.
   b. Understand and explore the issues involved in professionalism as nurses.
   c. Accept the fact that nursing is a profession.
   d. Cross-train with other health care providers such as physical therapist, laboratory technicians, and radiologist.

10. Power that originates in the ability to punish is called:
    a. Coercive
    b. Reward
    c. Legitimate
    d. Referent

11. Power that originates in a legal act is called:
    a. Coercive.
    b. Reward
    c. Legitimate
    d. Referent

12. Which of the following would be important for determining a profession from the power approach to professions?
    a. The members of the profession attain all the traits required for that profession.
    b. The members of the profession have high income levels.
    c. The profession is near the end of its developmental process.
    d. The education for the member of the professions must be attained in graduate schools.

13. A group of tasks assigned to one individual best describes:

   a. Position

   b. Occupation

   c. Profession

   d. Stint

Answers

1-c	6-b	11-c
2-d	7-c	12-d
3-b	8-c	13-a
4-d	9-b	
5-b	10-a	

Additional Critical Thinking Exercises

1. Do you think that a baccalaureate degree is the necessary minimal educational requirement for professional nursing? Develop an argument that would convince nurses, politicians, and the public of your position.

2. Develop a plan for establishing a nationwide nurse support network. Include in your plan who should be in the network, how it should be organized and run, and how "new" nurses can be groomed for high level administrative positions.

3. Identify politicians who have a health care background. Which of these politicians are nurses?

4. Prepare a 15 minute presentation on the topic "Nurses, Power, and Professionalism" to be given to a local civic organization.

Student Handout

You have been appointed as a student representative to the curriculum committee assigned to identify and define the tasks expected of students at each level of their education.

	Nursing Knowledge	Professional Person	Care Giver	Coordinator of Care
Definition	Knowledge based on theory and learning from the psychologic, biologic, social sciences, and liberal arts.			
Freshman-Level Skills	Discuss the relationship of nursing theory to nursing practice			
Sophomore-Level Skills	Use theory and knowledge in describing professional nursing			
Junior-Level Skills	Develop client care plans based on nursing knowledge			
Senior-Level Skills	Use theory based care plans in the provision of nursing care.			
New Graduate-Level Level Skills	Use and evaluate client plans of care based on nursing knowledge			

Chapter 2: Theories and Models in Nursing

Chapter 2 presents fundamental background information about theories and models in nursing, why they are important to a profession, and how they can be used in client care. The four underlying concepts found in all nursing models are presented. A brief explanation of *Systems Theory*, along with some of the key terminology, is presented because it is the foundation for many of the mainstream nursing theories now in use. Six nursing models or theories are discussed in relationship to the four underlying concepts common to all.

Teaching Points

1. Identify the differences between theory and model, and stress why their development indicates maturing of the profession of nursing.
2. Present and discuss the four common elements found in all nursing theories, client, environmental and health, and nursing.
3. Discuss *Systems Theory*, defining the key concepts and terms. Point out why understanding systems theory is necessary for understanding nursing models.
4. Present one to all six nursing theories discussed in the chapter. Explore the underlying philosophy of the theory, the operational definition of each of the four common concepts, and the advantages and disadvantages of each theory.

Questions

1. A particular system has a high degree of nonsummativity. You would expect that:

    a. There is a low degree of interdependence of components.

    b. The system will go from the complex to the simple.

    c. Little exchange between the system and the environment will take place.

    d. There is a high degree of interdependence of components.

2. Most living organisms are considered to be:

    a. Open systems

    b. Closed systems

    c. Subsystems

    d. Macrosystems

3. In Roy's model for nursing, the major component for the maintenance of health is the concept of:

    a. Systems

    b. Lack of illness

    c. Adaptation

    d. Use of medicine

4. "Stimuli" in the Roy model is synonymous with which of the following elements in the systems theory?

    a. Output

    b. Feedback

    c. Input

    d. Coping

5. In the Roy model of nursing, health is described as:

    a. A continuum

    b. A lack of illness

    c. A state or process of being and becoming an integrated whole person

    d. A state of physical and mental well-being

6. The framework for assessment in the Roy model is based on which two concepts:

    a. Cognator and regulator

    b. Input and stimuli

    c. Output and behavioral responses

    d. Focal and contextual

7. The second level assessment modes are most closely related to which part of the system?

    a. Input

    b. Output

    c. Ventral system

    d. Feedback loop

8. Understanding and using a nursing theory or model in practice is important because:

    a. It aids the practitioner to provide his or her care in an organized manner

    b. It contributes to the "professionalism" of the practitioner and profession

    c. It helps in understanding the relationship of the parts to each other

    d.   All of the above

9.   Which four concepts are common in most nursing theories?
    a.   Client, health, environment, nursing
    b.   Care, adaptation, system, cure
    c.   Nurse, physician, client, other providers
    d.   Hospital, nursing home, clinic, physician's office

10.   Orem's Self-Care model is based on the belief that:
    a.   The nurse helps the client adapt to his or her illness.
    b.   Cure of the client is the primary goal of health care.
    c.   Health care is the responsibility of each individual.
    d.   Health care goals much be established for each client.

11.   In the Orem model, the goal of nursing is to:
    a.   Re-establish the absolute state of health the client had before
         his or her illness.
    b.   Help the client conduct self-care activities to reach the highest
         level of functioning.
    c.   Prevent further injury to the client's biosystems.
    d.   Help balance the technologic care with the humanistic aspects
         of care.

12.   A major contribution that the King model made to the practice of
    nursing is:
    a.   The formalization of the use of goals to guide client care
    b.   The introduction of the concept of care as a key element in
         nursing care
    c.   Use of the idea of adaptation as an important client goal

d.   The in integration of Systems Theory into nursing care

13.   One aspect of Watson's Human Caring model that distinguishes it
       from most other nursing models is:
       a.   Understanding health as a dynamic state rather than a static
              goal
       b.   Viewing nursing as a process to help clients achieve their
              greatest potential rather than a curing profession
       c.   Use of a philosophical approach rather than a systems theory
              approach
       d.   Defining environment as both internal and external rather than
              just external

14.   Which of the following would be considered important aspects of
       caring according to the Watson model?
       a.   Establishing a helping-trusting relationship
       b.   Manipulating the environment to make it supportive
       c.   Assisting as necessary to meet the basic human needs of the
              client
       d.   All of the above

15.   Which of the following would be the most accurate description of
       "client" in the Johnson model?
       a.   An individual who is responsible for his or her own health
              care
       b.   A behavioral system that is an integrated whole
       c.   A dynamic entity with both input and output
       d.   An individual who must adapt to illness

16. The Neuman Health-Care Systems model is:

    a. Based solely on systems theory

    b. Appropriate only for nurses and nursing

    c. Nurse centered rather than client centered

    d. Applicable to a variety of health care disciplines

17. One of the key functions of the nurse in Neuman Model is to:

    a. Identify at what level a disruption in the client's internal stability has taken place.

    b. Return the client to a state of adaptation.

    c. Set goals for the fulfillment of client needs.

    d. Assist the client to reach his or her greatest potential.

Answers

1-d	7-b	13-c
2-a	8-d	14-d
3-c	9-1	15-b
4-c	10-c	16-d
5-c	11-b	17-a
6-a	12-a	

Additional Critical Thinking Exercises

1. What role does nursing theory play in the development of nursing as a unique health care profession?
2. What are the similarities and differences between nursing research and nursing theory?
3. Have the student select a client they have been assigned to during their clinical practice, and analyze that client's care according to a nursing model.
4. Are all nursing theories perfect? Select three of the presented theories and analyze them for strengths and weaknesses.

Student Handout Develop your own nursing theory using the following format:

Belief About:	Definition	Theory
Health		
Environment		
Client		
Nursing		

Chapter 3: Nursing Process, Critical Thinking, Nursing Dx

In Chapter 3, the concept of *critical thinking* is introduced as an essential element in the practice of nursing. The ways critical thinking can be and is used in nursing are discussed. The four steps of the critical thinking process are outlined and related to the nursing process. Nursing process is then presented as a client health care problem-solving approach with a discussion of its importance in providing professional level nursing care. The five steps of the nursing process are outlined in detail. The chapter concludes with information about nursing diagnosis, how it differs from medical diagnosis, and how it is used in providing nursing care.

Teaching Points

1. Introduce the concept of critical thinking, explain what it is, how and why it is important to professional nursing.
2. Explain the purpose of the nursing process. Present and define its five parts and demonstrate how it can be used in client care.
3. Stress how and why nursing diagnosis is different from medical diagnosis.

Questions

1. The first step in the process of critical thinking is:
    a. Identify the underlying beliefs.
    b. Identify the problem.
    c. Identify the value systems conflicts.
    d. Identify the best solution to the conflict.

2.	Which of the following is the most accurate statement about a nurse's value system?

	a.	Nurses must learn to disregard the value systems of the clients they work with to provide the best care.

	b.	The nurse's value system must be set aside when working with clients who have different value systems.

	c.	Nurses must adapt and change their value systems to conform with the value systems of the clients being cared for.

	d.	The nurse's personal value system influences how situations are perceived and what decisions are made.

3.	Which of the following are the best sources of support for beliefs?

	a.	Opinions and stereotypes

	b.	News programs and documentaries

	c.	Written reports and published surveys

	d.	Discussions and informal feedback from clients

4.	Biases are defined as:

	a.	Documented beliefs

	b.	Confirmation of facts

	c.	Information consistent with reality

	d.	Unjustified personal opinions and prejudices

5. An important role that the nursing process fulfills in professional nursing is to:

   a. Identify specific nursing actions for which nurses can be held publicly accountable.

   b. Distinguish nursing care from medical care.

   c. Prevent nurses from making errors in care that can lead to malpractice suits.

   d. Form the ethical basis for nursing practice.

6. Which of the following is the LAST step in the nursing process?

   a. Planning

   b. Evaluation

   c. Analysis

   d. Implementation

7. Which of the following would constitute information gather through the assessment step in the nursing process?

   a. Description of symptoms

   b. Laboratory test values

   c. Information from other health care providers

   d. All of the above

8. What differentiates nursing diagnosis from medical diagnosis?

   a. Nursing diagnosis is based on information gathered from the assessment of the client.

   b. Medical diagnosis identifies client care problems that affect the whole client.

   c. Nursing diagnosis identifies client problems that nurses can treat independently.

d. There is no difference between medical and nursing diagnosis.

9. The planning step in the nursing process always begins with:
   a. Formulation and establishment of goals or outcomes for the client
   b. Collection of all the data available about the client's condition
   c. Prioritizing the steps of the nursing care to be provided
   d. Writing down the nursing diagnosis

10. If all of the following goals were appropriate for a client, which would have the highest priority?
    a. Prevent injury from falls due to confusion.
    b. Re-establish role as primary provider for the family.
    c. Improve body image after leg amputation.
    d. Control postoperative bleeding.

11. What needed to be established before evaluation became a formal and organized part of the nursing process?
    a. Nursing models and theories
    b. Updated state practice acts for nurses
    c. Standards of care
    d. Managed care institutions

12. "Problems that the client is at risk for developing" best describes:
    a. Actual problems
    b. Possible problems
    c. Potential problems
    d. Likely problems

13. If all the following nursing diagnosis are appropriate for a client in an automobile accident, which one would have the highest priority?

    a.   Altered cerebral tissue perfusion

    b.   Disturbance in body image

    c.   Impaired home maintenance management

    d.   Dysfunctional grieving

14. Which is the most important aspect of the implementation step of the nursing process?

    a.   Providing care that meets the standards of care

    b.   Meeting all the care goals by the end of the shift

    c.   Involving the client as much as possible in the provision of care

    d.   Preventing the client from helping with the care since it is the nurse's responsibility

15. Which of the following is a FALSE statement about nursing diagnosis?

    a.   It is concerned with both health and illness.

    b.   It forms the basis for selecting certain nursing interventions.

    c.   It is a clinical judgment about individuals, families, or the community.

    d.   It is only acceptable when one of the approved NANDA nursing diagnosis is used.

Answers

1-b	5-a	9-a	13-a
2-d	6-c	10-d	14-c
3-c	7-d	11-c	15-d
4-d	8-c	12-c	

Additional Critical Thinking Exercises

1.   The following two case studies provide examples of failures in nursing care that resulted in injuries to patients and law suits.

    a.   Have the students discuss these two case studies and how the use of the nursing process would have prevented the incidents from occurring.

    b.   Have the students develop a care plan for each patient in the case studies that would include measures to prevent the injuries from   occurring

CASE STUDY

A nurse was sued for failure to take appropriate nursing action when she improperly administered a tube feeding. It was towards the end of the shift when the nurse remembered that she had to give a client a tube feeding. In a hurry to get home, she did not check the position of the tube prior to the administration of the feeding. She poured the feeding rapidly into the nasogastric feeding tube, and continued to do so even though the feeding fluid was coming out of the client's nose and mouth, and he was gagging and in respiratory distress. Despite the client's distress, the nurse left the room and went home. An orderly came into the room after report and sought assistance for the client who was now unresponsive. The client died a short time later.

(Aiken, TD: Legal, Ethical, and Political Issues In Nursing. FA Davis: Philadelphia, 1995.)

CASE STUDY

Failure to communicate lead to a $1 million jury judgment against a nurse in Maine. The client had returned to the recovery room from surgery for the removal of a foreign object lodged in his esophagus. At about one hour post-op, the client's wife reported to the recovery room nurse that her husband was wheezing and in pain. The nurse recognized these symptoms as indicative of an esophageal tear, but did not notify the surgeon of the client's condition for six hours. When the surgeon was finally notified of the client's condition, the client was taken back to surgery and a corrective procedure was performed. Unfortunately, the client's esophagus had become infected with organisms from his GI tract during the 6-hour period before the tear was repaired, and he died shortly after. His wife brought a law suit against the hospital for negligence on the part of the nurse. The court ruled that the nurse's failure to promptly notify the surgeon was a failure to follow a standard of care.

(Aiken, TD: <u>Legal, Ethical, and Political Issues In Nursing.</u> FA Davis: Philadelphia 1995.)

2.   Have the students work in pairs. After obtaining a health history from each other, have the students use the steps in the nursing process to prepare a nursing care plan for the other student based on his or her health needs. They should include three nursing diagnosis in this plan.

Chapter 4: The Process of Educating Nurses

Chapter 4 begins with a presentation of the history and development of nursing education throughout the ages. It discusses the current types of nursing education found in the United States, including hospital based diploma programs, baccalaureate education, practical nursing, and associated degree programs. Advanced level nursing including master's, doctorate, and advanced practice programs are outlined. The ANA Position Paper on Education for Nursing is presented with an analysis of current nursing education practices and implications for the future of nursing education.

Teaching Points

1. Interrelate current educational practices in nursing with their historical developments. Point out which strengths and weakness in current nursing education can be traced to their historical basis.
2. Discuss the various types of educational programs available for nurses. Which are professional? Which are technical?
3. Describe the advanced degree preparation that are open to nurses. What do these prepare the nurse to do that is different from the basic program?
4. Present the ANA Position Paper on Nursing Education. Explain what it means to current nursing education practices and what changes are required in nursing education to meet its goals.

Questions

1. A type of nursing education program which is conducted in junior or community. colleges that is nominally two years in length is:

   a. Diploma program

   b. Baccalaureate program

   c. Associate Degree Program

   d. Professional nursing program

2. An important similarity among the various types of educational programs for nurses is:

   a. Homogeneity of entering students

   b. No state or national approval is required

   c. The same courses are taught in all programs

   d. Clinical experience is required to gain certain knowledge and skills

3. An important element found in baccalaureate nursing programs and not in other types of nursing educations programs is:

   a. Development of the total intellectual skills of the individual

   b. The use of nursing theory and models in developing practice

   c. Learning the basic skills and principles involved in teaching and management

   d. All of the above

4. Which of the following was the most significant contribution of Florence Nightingale to nursing education?

   a. Recognizing that formal, systematic education in both theory and practice was essential for the preparation of high quality nurses.

   b. Advocating that all nurses be educated in universities so that nursing care would meet the standards established by the government.

   c. Forcing physicians and hospitals to recognize that clinical practice was not as important as the theory-based learning obtained in the classroom.

   d. Enforcing the requirement that all nursing instructors have a master's degree in nursing to provide the highest quality education possible for students.

5. Which of the following best describes nursing education in the United States during the 1800s and early 1900s?

   a. It was high quality with a balance between classroom education and clinical practice.

   b. Strict criteria were established for nursing education by the NLN and the ANA to guarantee high quality education.

   c. There was no formal nursing education programs during this time period; nurses were trained in apprenticeships only.

   d. There was little or no classroom education and students learned by hands-on experience during their 12 to 14 hour shifts on the hospital units.

6. What was a major benefit of the diploma type training programs for nurses?

   a. Nurses from these programs were assertive and could stand-up to physicians who made unrealistic demands.

   b. Nurses from diploma programs were proficient in basic nursing skills and could assume a hospital position with minimal orientation.

   c. Nurses trained in diploma programs were often limited to employment in the institutions where they were trained.

   d. All diploma schools were regulated by the NLN criteria and met strict standards for educating students.

7. State boards of nursing were concerned most about which of the following practices found in many diploma programs?

   a. Excessive use of classroom time during the program

   b. Mandatory housing of the students in a closed dormitory near the hospital

   c. Use of the students as unpaid hospital personnel while in their education programs

   d. The high failure rates of diploma graduates on the NCLEX examinations

8. *Career ladder* in education refers to:

   a. Specialized programs for associate degree or diploma RNs to attain a baccalaureate degree.

   b. The ability of staff nurses to be promoted based on their clinical skills.

   c. The relationship between one level of nursing education to the next higher level of education.

d.   The fact that once nurses pass the NCLEX examination they are all considered professionals.

9.   Which of the following are common characteristics of LPN educational programs?

a.   Located on college campus, two years in length, require no clinical experiences

b.   Theory oriented curriculum, wide scope of practice, highly selective admission

c.   Technically oriented, located in votec or community colleges, 9 to 12 months in length

d.   All of the above

10.   Which of the following are considered *advanced practice nurses*?

a.   Family nurse practitioner

b.   Renal clinical nurse specialist

c.   Nurse midwife

d.   All of the above

11.   The main position advocated by the ANA Position Paper on Education for Nurses is that:

a.   Any nursing education program is acceptable as long as the graduates take and pass the NCLEX examination.

b.   Baccalaureate education should be the basic level of preparation for professional nurses.

c.   Associate degree education should be the basic level of preparation for professional nurses.

d.   Only nurses educated at the master degree or higher level should be considered professional nurses.

12. Which of the following is the most important consequence of the ANA Position Paper on Education for Nurses?

    a. Increased numbers of associate degree programs

    b. Large numbers of students graduating with baccalaureate degrees in nursing

    c. Resistance to the proposal by hospitals and diploma nursing programs

    d. Demand for a clear distinction between technical and professional nursing programs

13. Requirements for entry into a master degree nursing program usually include:

    a. Baccalaureate degree in nursing

    b. At least one year of experience as an RN

    c. Satisfactory score on the GRE or MAT

    d. All of the above

Answers

1-c	6-b	11-b
2-d	7-c	12-d
3-d	8-a	13-d
4-a	9-c	
5-d	10-d	

Additional Critical Thinking Exercises

1.   Have the students interview three RNs with different educational backgrounds (BS, AD, Diploma). Include in the interview how adequately the nurse feels she or he was prepared for practice, how their work has changed, and if they feel the need for more education.

2.   Working in groups, the students can survey several health care facilities in their region that hire RNs. Do the facilities differentiate between the different levels of education by nurses? Are there any rewards for having a BS degree over an AD or diploma?

3.   In group discussion, compare the concepts of technical and professional nursing practice as it is defined by the ANA. Obtain copies of job descriptions and qualifications for staff nurses at several facilities. Do these reflect the different levels of nursing? How?

Student Handout

STUDENT JOB DESCRIPTION

Assess, plans and implements the nursing process and when assigned directs others in the implementation of the plan of care in accordance with the State Nurse Practice Act and ANA Code for Nurses.

JOB STANDARDS

1. Performs and documents patient, family, and or community assessments with consideration of biophysical, psychosocial, environmental, self care, educational, and discharge planning factors.

    PR: 3,6,9,10,11,12,13,14,15,16,17,18,19,20.

    Measurement Method: Documentation, observation reported variances.

2. Coordinates and provides care for a patient or a group of assigned patients in a safe, effective manner.

    PR:3,6,9,10,11,12,13,14,15,16,17,18,19,20.

    Daily plans, coordinates, delegates, and provides care based on standards of practice and standards of patient care that reflect the stated diagnosis, patient care needs, problems, or knowledge deficits based on the patient assessment.

    Measurement Method: Documentation, observation, reported variances

3. Collaborates with other members of the health care team to assist in the plan of care.

    PR:3,14,15,16,18,

    Communicates with health care team in a neat, legible, organized, and accurate manner. The interventions implemented are relevant to the patient's identified care needs or knowledge deficits.

    Measurement Method: Documentation in patient records, observation, reported variances.

4. Evaluates patient care given by self and team members working with and under supervision.

   PR: 3,14,15,16,18

   Documents outcomes of nursing interventions including patient's responses to nursing interventions.

   Measurement Method: Documentation, observation, reported variances.

5. Evaluates patient's and/or family's knowledge of disease process and intervenes and educates patients and significant others as appropriate.

   PR: 3,14,15,16,18

   Evaluates effectiveness of teaching plan by documenting methods and patient and significant other's understanding of teaching plan. Also evaluates the understanding of teaching as demonstrated by patient and significant other.

   Measurement Method: Documentation, observation, reported variances.

6. Prepares patient for discharge.

   PR: 3,6,9,10,11,12,13,14,15,16,17,18,19,20

   Ensures continuing care needs are assessed and referrals for such care are documented in the medical record.

7. Cares for patients and/or families in community settings.

   PR: 3,14,15,16,18

   Documents assessment of client/environment interaction, implements appropriate interventions under supervision.

8. Continues professional growth and development through attendance and active participation in classroom activities, professional affiliations, inservice, seminars, workshops, conferences, and continuing education.

   PR: 3,14,15,16,18

Attends all classes regularly and is prepared for clinical assignments. Maintains CPR certification and immunization status. Keeps current on infection control, safety, and hazardous substances.
Measurement Method: Documentation.

9.   Performs other student nursing duties as directed. Participates in departmental committees or activities; presents inservice, programs or performs other assignments.
Measurement Method: Documentation.

DIRECTORY OF PHYSICAL REQUIREMENTS

PR1: Lifting, pushing, pulling, carrying or otherwise moving 10 pounds maximum and occasionally lifting and/or carrying such articles as files, ledgers, and small tools. Although a sedentary job is defined as one that involves sitting, a certain amount of walking, standing and/or mobility is often necessary in carrying out job duties. **SEDENTARY WORK CLASS**

PR2: Lifting, pushing, pulling, carrying or otherwise moving 20 pounds maximum with frequent lifting and/or carrying of objects weighing up to 10 pounds. Even though the weight lifted may be only a negligible amount, a job is in this category when it requires walking, standing and/or mobility to a significant degree of pushing and pulling of arm and/or leg controls. **LIGHT WORK CLASS**

PR3: Lifting, pushing, pulling, carrying or otherwise moving 50 pounds maximum with frequent lifting and/or carrying of objects weighing up to 25 pounds. **MEDIUM WORK CLASS.**

PR4: Lifting, pushing, pulling, carrying or otherwise moving 100 pounds maximum with frequent lifting and/or carrying of objects weighing up to 50 pounds. **HEAVY WORK CLASS.**

PR5: Lifting, pushing, pulling, carrying or otherwise moving objects in excess of 100 pounds with frequent lifting and/or carrying of objects weighing up to 50 pounds. **VERY HEAVY WORK CLASS.**

PR6: Walking/standing 80% or above of scheduled work shift.

PR7: Climbing: ascending/descending ladders, stairs, and so on using feet/legs and/or hands/arms.

PR8: Balancing: maintaining body equilibrium to prevent falling when sitting, walking, standing, crouching, or running.

PR9:   a. Stooping: bending the body downwards and forward by bending the spine at the waist.

       b. Kneeling: bending the legs at the knees to come to rest on the knee or knees.

       c. Crouching: bending the body downward and forward by bending the legs and spine.

       d. Crawling: moving about on the hands and knees or hands and feet.

PR10: Reaching: extending the hands and arms in any direction.

PR11: Handling: seizing, holding, grasping, turning, or otherwise working with the hand or hands (fingering not involved). **MANUAL DEXTERITY.**

PR12: Fingering: picking pinching or otherwise working with the fingers primarily (rather than with the whole hand or arms as in handling). **FINGER DEXTERITY.**

PR13: Feeling: perceiving such attributes of object/materials as size, shape, temperature, texture, movement, or pulsation by receptors in the skin, particularly those of the finger tips.

PR14: Talking: expressing and exchanging ideas by means of the spoken word.

PR15: Hearing: perceiving the nature of sounds by the ear, discerning and understanding the human voice and hearing auscultatory sounds.

PR16: a. Acuity, far: clarity of vision at 20 feet or more
      b. Acuity, near: clarify of vision at 20 inches or less

PR17: Depth perception: three dimensional vision. The ability to judge distance and space relationships so as to see objects where and as they actually are.

PR18: Field of vision: the area that can be seen up and down or to the right or left while the eyes are fixed on a given point.

PR19: Accommodation: adjustment of the lens of the eye to bring an object into sharp focus especially important for near-point work at varying distances from the eye.

PR20: Color vision: the ability to identity and distinguish colors.

Chapter 5: Ethics in Nursing

In Chapter 5, the student is initiated into the language and concepts of professional ethics as it applies to health care and nursing. An initial section on definition of common terms used in ethics is followed by a brief presentation of the important ethical concepts that underlay most ethical dilemmas the student is likely to encounter in practice. Two commonly used ethical systems are outlined and explained, stressing their strengths and weaknesses. The ANA Code of Ethics is presented. The chapter also includes an ethical decision making model based on the nursing process and a discussion of the nature of ethical dilemmas.

Teaching Points

1. Discuss ethics as an important element of nursing and health care, indicating that it has its own specialized language and use of terms. Define the terms.
2. Define and give examples for each of the important ethical concepts.
3. Present the two ethical systems of Utilitarianism and Deontology. Point out there advantages and disadvantages, and demonstrate how they can be used to make ethical decisions.
4. Outline the steps for the ethical decision making model. Give examples of when and how this can be used in client care situations.

Questions

1. Concepts, ideals, behaviors, and significant themes that give meaning to a person's life best describes:
   a. Morals
   b. Values
   c. Laws
   d. Ethics

2. Rules of conduct that protect the social fabric are known as:
   a. Morals
   b. Values
   c. Laws
   d. Ethics

3. Standards of right and wrong that are often based on religious beliefs are otherwise known as:
   a. Morals
   b. Values
   c. Laws
   d. Ethics

4. Systems of valued behaviors and beliefs are:
   a. Morals
   b. Values
   c. Laws
   d. Ethics

5. Professional autonomy is always associated with:

   a. Legal immunity

   b. Decrease in work load

   c. Ethical accountability

   d. Ethical freedom

6. An ethical code can best be described as:

   a. A framework for decision making

   b. A collection of static rules

   c. A group of values legally binding

   d. The "ball and chain" of the profession

7. A system of ethical decision making that has as its focus a concern for efficiency and utility is called:

   a. Deontological

   b. Jurisditial

   c. Teleological

   d. Theological

8. Statement number two of the Ethical Code for Nurses states: "The nurse safeguards the client's right to privacy by judiciously protecting information of a confidential nature." This statement is based on:

   a. The principle that the right to privacy is an inalienable right of all persons

   b. The fact that the nurse-client relationship is based on trust

   c. The fact that an inappropriate breach of confidentiality may expose the nurse to liability

   d. All of the above

9.   In comparing the ethical code for nurses to the law, it is an accurate statement to say:

   a.   If a law is not broken, then the nurse is following the ethical code.

   b.   If the ethical code and the law have a discrepancy, it is always better to follow the law.

   c.   The ethical code encompasses all the pertinent laws.

   d.   All of the above are accurate statements.

10.   Which of the following is not a characteristic of an ethical code:

   a.   It is "action oriented"

   b.   It is a set of static rules

   c.   It is a written list of the values of the profession

   d.   It is used in day-to-day decision making

11.   A system of ethical decision making that is based on the "greatest good" principle, is called:

   a.   Egoism

   b.   Utilitarianism

   c.   Deontological

   d.   None of the above

12.   A system of ethical decision making based on the discovery and confirmation of a set of morals or rules that govern the ethical dilemma is called:

   a.   Deontological

   b.   Jurisdictional

   c.   Teleological

   d.   Theological

13. The ethical principle requiring that the primary goal of health care and nursing is to do good for others is called:

    a. Autonomy

    b. Fidelity

    c. Beneficence

    d. Veracity

14. The ethical principle of nonmaleficence is defined as:

    a. Eealth care workers avoiding harm to patients

    b. Telling the truth to patients in all matters

    c. Being faithful to commitments made to patients

    d The right of self-determination of patients

15. When an ethical situation arises where there is a choice between two equally unfavorable alternatives, it is called:

    a. Tort

    b. Ethical antagonism

    c. Contraindication

    d. Ethical dilemma

16. The first step in the ethical decision making process is to:

    a Consider the alternatives

    b. Collect, analyze and interpret the data

    c. Consider the consequences of the actions

    d. Make a decision

Answers

1-b	7-c	13-c
2-c	8-b	14-a
3-a	9-c	15-d
4-d	10-b	16-b
5-c	11-b	
6-a	12-a	

CASE STUDY

A 24 year old part-time housekeeper finds out that she is pregnant for the third time. She has ended both previous pregnancies with abortions. She has been living with a man who physically abuses her and has decided to leave him. She has recently joined a church that strongly opposes abortion and emphasizes that the woman's role is one that is subservient to men. Her job pays too little to support a baby by herself, and she refuses to go on welfare. Her family has cut her off since she started living with her boyfriend, and she has no other support systems. How should the nurse in the public health care clinic counsel this woman in making a decision about her pregnancy?

CASE STUDY

A mentally retarded woman has a baby with multiple birth defects and congenital abnormalities. Because she is unable to take care of the infant, the child is placed in a state run hospital with a court appointed legal guardian. The primary physician assigned to the infant believes in very aggressive treatment for all his clients, and outlines a course of treatment that includes several complex and expensive operations over a period of several years. The child will be spending most of the first several years of his life in the intensive care unit at great expense, borne by the hospital and state, with no guarantee that any of the treatments will help. What type of decision about this child's care should be made? Who should make these decisions?

CASE STUDY - WHEN THE PATIENT REFUSES CARE

Bill Z, a 6 foot 3 inch, 135 lbs, 76 year old retired college professor was admitted to a medical unit in a large metropolitan hospital. He had been diagnosed six months previously as having metastatic cancer that had spread from his lungs, to the liver, GI system, and bones. He had received some chemotherapy but with will little effect. He was admitted to the hospital because he had become too weak to walk or care for himself at home, and because the large doses of oral narcotic medications were having little effect on his generalized pain.

His physician had decided that further chemotherapy would be useless, and ordered that Mr. Z was to be kept comfortable with medications. A continuous morphine sulfate intravenous drip was started to help control the pain. Although talkative and friendly by nature, as Mr. Z's cancer spread, he would cry out and beg the nurses not to move him. Because he was very tall and underweight, his bony prominences quickly became reddened and show signs of breakdown. The hospital standards of care for bed ridden clients required that they be turned from side to side every two hours. Mr. Z yelled so loudly when he was turned that he nursing staff wondered if they were helping him or hurting him.

To decide what should be done, a client care conference was called by the nurses most often involved in providing care for Mr. Z. The head nurse of the unit stated very clearly that the hospital standards of care required that he be turned at least every two hours to prevent skin breakdown, infections, and perhaps sepsis. In his already weakened condition, an infection or sepsis would most likely be fatal. Rebecca F, who had been an RN for some 15 years disagreed with the head nurse. Her feeling was that causing this obviously terminal client as much pain as he was having by turning him was cruel and violated his dignity as a human being. She stated that she could not stand to hear him yell any more and refused to take care of him until some other decision was made about his nursing care. Susan B, a new graduate nurse felt that the patient should have some say in his own care and that perhaps some type of compromise could be reached about turning him, even if less frequently. Ellen R, who had worked on the unit for two years, felt that the physician should make the decision on turning this client and then all the nurses would have to do was follow the order. This last suggestion was met with strong negative comments by the other nurses present. They felt that client comfort and turning are nursing measures.

What should they decide? Violation of a standard of care can leave a nurse open to a law suit. What about the client's right to decide when it violates a standard of care? Are there ever any situations when a nurse might legally and ethically violate a standard of care? What are the consequences? (Aiken, TD: Legal, Ethical, and Political Issues In Nursing FA Davis, Philadelphia 1995.)

Additional Critical Thinking Exercises

1. Define *Utilitarianism* and list its advantages and disadvantages as an ethical decision making system.

2. Define *Deontology* and list its advantages and disadvantages as an ethical decision making system.

3. Divide the class into 11 equal groups, and assign each group one of the ethical principles found in the ANA Code. Have them present a case study (real or fictional) that illustrates the statement.

4. Using one of the case studies above, or any of the case studies presented in the book, have the students apply the ethical decision making process to the case study and offer possible resolutions for it.

5.   Susan had worked as an aid for five years at a nursing home when she enrolled in an associate degree nursing program. She continued to work at the nursing home part-time while she completed the program and became an RN. After graduation, the nursing home offered Susan a position as director, while a large medical center in a distant city offered her a position in their rehabilitation unit. All Susan's family, and her boyfriend, live in the same city as the nursing home. Use a value clarification process to make a choice about Susan's career.

Values Clarification Exercise

PART I. - Rank the following from 1 to 5, with one being the item with the highest priority, and 5 being the item with lowest priority.

A.   A hospital must cut back its budget or go bankrupt. Which of the following clients should be given priority for care?

_____ A newborn infant with multiple birth defects who is likely to be retarded for life

_____ A 47 year old male scientist with an acute MI who has just discovered a new medication that might cure HIV

_____ An 88 year old retired female grade school teacher who was recently diagnosed with liver cancer

_____ A 17 year old runaway who is addicted to cocaine and is pregnant

_____ A 58 year old construction worker who has severe emphysema due to his 2.5 pack a day smoking habit

B.   The nurse is assigned to a client who has a bleeding ulcer secondary to stress. Which aspects of his care would receive highest priority?

_____ Give him pain medications to make him comfortable.

_____ Explain the relationship between stress and ulcers.

_____ Involve him as much as possible in his self-care.

_____ Encourage him to talk about his job, family, and so on.

_____ Teach him about diet and medication to control ulcers.

45

PART II. - Rate the following statements on a scale of 1 to 5 (1=strongly support; 2=support; 3=no opinion; 4=reject; 5=strongly reject)

1. Abortion is always wrong, no matter what the circumstances..._____

2. People who receive the death penalty deserve it ...._____

3. Life support should be terminated for clients when they are not likely to live ...._____

4. Street drugs should be made legal ...._____

5. Prisoners, genetically defective persons and mentally retarded persons should be sterilized..........................._____

6. Premature, drug addicted newborns should be allowed to die..._____

7. Condoms should be given out in high schools to prevent pregnancy and HIV..._____

8. All hospitalized clients should be routinely screened for HIV, and AIDS ...._____

9. Scientists should be allowed to use aborted fetuses for fetal tissue research..._____

10. All newborn infants should be genetically screened for inherited diseases ...._____

PART III. - Complete the following sentences.

1. The one thing I have always wanted to do is_____.

2. If I just inherited 5 million dollars, I would_____.

3. As president of the United States, I would_____.

4. If I died today, I would like my obituary to say_____ .

5. If I could control the world and its destiny, I would_____.

PART IV. - Below is a partial list of things people value.

Complete the list, then rank each item from 1 (highest value) to 8 (lowest value)

_____family   _____

_____career   _____

_____religion   _____

_____honor   _____

_____material possessions   _____

_____health   _____

_____recreation   _____

____professionalism   _____

Ask the students what they learned about themselves by doing this exercise. What do the ranking signify? Can the students identify themselves as more utilitarian, or more deontological?

How do they feel about their ethical standards? High, average or low?

Chapter 6: Bioethical Issues

Chapter 6 presents some of the bioethical issues found in today's health care system. Through an analysis of each topic, the students are introduced to the underlying dilemmas that are associated with such issues as abortion, genetic research, fetal tissue experimentation, organ transplantation, use of scarce resources, assisted suicide, and AIDS. Information is included about the importance of being an organ donor, and the proper way to formulate a living will.

Teaching Points

1. Discuss abortion including the ethical aspects of nurses who work with abortion clients, the implications of Roe vs. Wade decision, and the nurses right to refuse to participate.
2. Present the ethical issues that are involved in genetic research, particularly the idea of confidentiality.
3. Include the potential abuses of fetal tissue research if there are no controls on its use.
4. Stress the issue of informed consent (self-determination) and the selection process used for selecting organ recipients. Include a discussion of how the process takes place and the importance of being an organ donor.
5. Introduce the use of scarce resources ethical issue by describing the current state of health care in the United States. Use examples of high cost procedures and treatments that have little long-term benefits.
6. Discuss the underlying ethical issues involved in the HIV/AIDS question, including right
    to privacy, use of scarce resources, and right to care.

Questions

1. According to the Roe vs. Wade decision, abortion is:

    a.   Both moral and ethical

    b.   A right guaranteed by the Constitution of the United States

    c.   Included under the right to self-determination

    d.   A conflict between the rights of the mother and the rights of the fetus

2. The deontological school of ethics says that abortion:

    a.   Is the greatest good for the greatest number of individuals and therefore is ethical

    b.   Involves the conflicts of the right of the mother to self-determination with the right of the fetus to life

    c.   Can be performed for any reason because the law makes it legal and ethical

    d.   Can be performed in situations where the mother is unwed and already has several other children

3. From the teleological standpoint, abortion:

    a.   Is ethical only when the mother is pregnant due to rape or incest

    b.   Is never allowed for any reason due to the violation of the rights of the fetus

    c.   Can be performed anytime if the mother wants it

    d.   May or may not be ethical dependent on the issues and circumstances that Surround the individual situation

4. The major ethical considerations involved in genetic research revolve around the issues of:

    a. Production of abnormal and mutant organisms

    b. Violations of confidentiality and informed consent

    c. Breading of a "super-race" of humans due to purification of genetic material

    d. Loss of control of reproduction by the human species

5. Which of the following would be important for the nurse to assure when assisting in genetic screening procedures, such as amniocentesis?

    a. Informed consent is given freely by the client.

    b. The client understands the nature of the procedure.

    c. The client understands the type of information that will be produced by the procedure.

    d. All of the above.

6. A 9 month old baby who is developmentally delayed is tested for genetic abnormalities. After the results are back from the laboratory, a representative from the client's medical insurance company calls the nurses' station on the phone, and asks for the results of the tests. The nurse's best response to this request is to:

    a. Refuse to give the information over the phone.

    b. Give a noncommittal response that "everything is normal" even though it is untrue.

    c. Give the results as they are reported on the lab sheet because the insurance company is paying for the tests anyway.

    d. Tell the representative that the tests are not back yet.

7. A nurse who works in a federally funded abortion clinic becomes aware of the fact that aborted second trimester fetuses are being sent to a nearby university for research and transplantation. What should this nurse do with this knowledge?

    a. Keep quiet about the finding because she might loose her job.

    b. Confront the medical director of the clinic that this practice is both illegal and unethical.

    c. Tell her supervisor that she knows about what is going on and ask for a raise.

    d. Report the practice the Department of Health and Human Services.

8. The two most important ethical issues involved in organ transplantation are:

    a. Beneficence and nonmaleficence

    b. Self-determination and distributive justice

    c. Veracity and informed consent

    d. Fidelity and option rights

9. A 16 year old male client brought in to the emergency room with a gunshot wound to the head is declared brain dead. His driver's license identifies him as an organ donor, but the hospital staff is unable to locate his family for permission to take his organs. Another client in the same hospital will die within 24 hours without a heart transplant. The tissues of both clients match sufficiently for a transplant. What is the ethical course of action in this case?

    a. Take the donor's organs per permission of his driver's license.

    b. The organs cannot be taken without the family's permission because the client is under aged.

c. Continue to attempt to locate the client's family while preparing for the transplant.

d. Remove only those organs that will not kill the client.

10. An unresponsive 94 year old female client, who has recently had a leg amputated for terminal cancer, develops renal failure. She has no living relatives. Although hemodialysis will prolong her life for several weeks to several months, her health care team is having difficulty deciding if it should be initiated. What is the key ethical issues involved in this dilemma?

a. Distributive justice

b. Veracity

c. Fidelity

d. Nonmaleficence

11. A client in the intensive care unit has a "Do not resuscitate order" (DNR) on his chart. The nurse caring for him recognizes that DNR orders:

a. May be given orally by the physician

b. Have no specific time limit

c. Protect the client's family from making difficult decisions

d. Must be written by the physician.

12. A physician writes a DNR order on a competent client. Which of the following individuals may give permission for this order?

a. The client's spouse

b. The client's only child

c. The client

d. All of the above

13. Which of the following treatment modalities would most likely be considered extraordinary?
    a. Intravenous fluids by subclavian catheter
    b. Oxygen by face mask at 60%
    c. Counter-pulsating intra-aortic balloon pump
    d. Chest tubes

14. The practice of allowing a client to die without the use of any extraordinary measures is sometimes called:
    a. Active euthanasia
    b. Passive euthanasia
    c. Mercy killing
    d. Assisted suicide

15. Two important ethical issues that surround the HIV and AIDS client are:
    a. Confidentiality and right to care
    b. Self-determination and distributive justice
    c. Veracity and informed consent
    d. Fidelity and option rights

Answers

1-c	6-a	11-d
2-b	7-d	12-c
3-d	8-b	13-c
4-b	9-c	14-b
5-d	10-a	15-a

CASE STUDY

Four years ago, Wyman F was diagnosed as being positive for the LTM virus (this is a fictitious virus invented for the purpose of this case study). After a second test confirmed the diagnosis, he began the standard medical treatment for the disease, including frequent blood tests at the immune clinic where a great deal of research was being conducted into the transmission, prevention, progression, and treatment of the disease. At the time he started treatment, Mr. F signed the standard consent form for treatment, and a special consent form to be part of the ongoing research at the clinic. Approximately three years after treatment began, Mr. F's body began producing an unusual type of white blood cell that eventually destroyed the LTM virus rendering him completely free of the disease. Needless to say, the researchers at the clinic were very interested in this development, and saw in it a possible cure for the disease.

The physician-researcher at the clinic told Mr. F that he would have to return once a month to have blood samples drawn to insure that the disease did not recur. Shannon O, an RN who counsels clients in the clinic, became aware of the fact that the blood being drawn from Mr. F on his monthly visits was being used, without his knowledge, to clone the white blood cells that seemed to destroy the LTM virus. When Shannon confronted the physician about the possible unethical nature of this research, he told her to mind her own business. He told Shannon that she was in counseling, and not research, and that she didn't really know what was going on. Besides, Mr. F. had signed the consent form for research four years ago.

Several weeks after this exchange, it was announced that the clinic was in the process of developing a cure for LTM based on a new type of white blood cell created in the laboratory. The commercial and financial implications of this finding were tremendous. Should Shannon tell Mr. F.

that it was his blood cells that were the basis for this cure? Do cloned blood cells belong to the client? Was the physician completely ethical in his approach to this research? Is a consent form valid forever, and for all types of research? What ethical principles are involved in this dilemma? Did the physician violate any ethical principles?

CASE STUDY

By any standards, Mr. Neal T. was a complicated client to care for. At age 72, he had a long history of COPD, coronary artery disease, three myocardial infarctions, liver disease secondary to alcoholism, and an amputated right arm from an automobile accident. He was admitted with renal failure, and placed on a medical surgical unit for the weekend. He was disoriented, and lethargic, but cooperative with most procedures and hospital routines.

Bethany H. one of the RNs on the unit, was assigned to supervise the care for Mr. T. during her 12 hour shift. Early in the morning, Mr. T's most recent ex-wife came in to visit and help with his AM care. Even though they had been divorced for ten years, they had remained close, and spent a great deal of time together. This former wife informed Bethany that Mr. T. had told her many times that if anything should happen to him, he didn't want to be kept alive with tubes and machines.

Later in the day, Mr. T's son and daughter by an earlier marriage, arrived from out-of-state. They had not seen their father in several years, and were appalled at how much he had deteriorated. They requested to speak to the physician about Mr. T's condition and prognosis, but his attending physician was off call for the weekend. The physician taking call did not feel familiar enough with the case to discuss it with them either on the phone or in person. The son and daughter told Bethany that they wanted every thing possible done for their father until they got a chance to talk to the attending physician.

Mr. T's condition deteriorated rapidly during the shift, and by mid-afternoon he was totally unresponsive, his blood pressure was 72/40, pulse rate 144, and he had not had any urine output for five hours. Bethany called the on-call physician to see about a DNR order based on Mr. T's former wife's account of what the patient had requested. The physician said that while a DNR order seemed appropriate for this terminal client, he wasn't sure he could give it because he did not know the client that well. He wanted to think about it some more. The physician did order some furosemide (Lasix), an increase in the IV rate, and some blood work.

Just before the end of Bethany's shift, Mr. T's former wife called to see how he was doing. When informed of his critical condition, she begged the nurse to let Mr. T go peacefully. As Bethany was on her way to Mr. T's room with some medication, he went into cardiac arrest. Should she call a code and begin CPR as the son and daughter had requested? Should she let Mr. T. go peacefully as his former wife had requested? What part does the physician's response play in the decision? What could have been done to avoid this dilemma?

CASE STUDY

A 22 year old victim of a car accident had a broken neck and was a quadriplegic. After many months in painful rehabilitation with little progress, he asked that he be allowed to die by starvation while receiving only basic physical care and pain medications in the hospital. The physician refused to honor the request, and ordered a feeding tube inserted to force feed the client and keep him alive. On what ethical principle did the physician base his decisions and actions? Should the nurse carry out an order that clearly seemed to violate the client's right to self-determination? What actions might the nurse have taken? What would be the possible consequences to these actions?

CASE STUDY

A small rural hospital with a four bed intensive care unit had two women cardiac arrest within a few minutes of each other. One was a 52 year old college professor with teenage children at home, the other was a 78 year old widow from a nursing home with advanced Alzheimer's disease. Because the hospital and unit were so small, only one code cart with a defibrillator was available with one RN and one LPN on duty at the time. The RN had to decide which client to resuscitate.   On what ethical principles could she base a decision? What should her decision be?

Additional Critical Thinking Exercises

1.   Have the students take one of the positions on abortion and defend it using an ethical theory they selected and the rationale for their position.
2.   What are other implications or possible results of unregulated gene and fetal tissue research? How might these be prevented?
3.   Analyze the above case studies using the ethical decision making model. What are some possible resolutions to these cases? What is the rationale behind them?
4.   Have the students list all the diseases, health care conditions, and injuries they can think of. Then ask them to rank them in order of those that should be paid for by the government from highest to lowest priority.

5. Ask the students if they have signed the back of their driver's licenses as organ donor? Have them give reasons why or why not. Is there a possibility they might change their minds?

Chapter 7, Reality Shock in the Workplace

In Chapter 7, the student is introduced to some of the realities of the workplace. The goal of the chapter is to help the student through the transition process by awareness of the problems that are involved. A discussion of the various roles for nurses that the student may encounter is presented. Several methods of lessening role transition shock are presented. The topic of burnout is presented, including symptoms of burnout, and methods to prevent it or deal with it. Time management techniques, good health practices, and stress reduction are discussed. The chapter also helps the student prepare for employment after graduation. It discusses career opportunities, preparing a resume, and conducting an employment interview.

Teaching Points

1. Present the definition of the different roles and indicate how conflict among these roles often form the basis of reality shock.
2. Discuss ways that the student can prevent or cope with reality shock.
3. Describe burnout, discuss the symptoms, and list some ways that it can be presented.
4. Describe the realities of the current work place and the realistic employment opportunities for nurses in today's health care system.
5. Indicate the important aspects of a well written resume, why it is important, and should be avoided.
6. List the elements in an employment interview, and give the student the do's and don'ts of such an interview.

Questions

1. What the nurse actually does while practicing nursing defines:

    a.   ideal role.

    b.   perceived role.

    c.   performed role.

    d.   practice role.

2. Unresolved role conflicts may result in:

    a.   high levels of anxiety.

    b.   physical symptoms.

    c.   emotional symptoms.

    d.   all of the above.

3. Which of the following is the most effective way for students to lessen role conflict?

    a.   Become involved in an internship between the junior and senior years in nursing school.

    b.   Avoid contact with nurses in the hospital because they have a very negative attitude.

    c.   Seek psychological counseling with qualified psychotherapist.

    d.   Discuss emotions and feelings about nursing school with other nursing students at least once a week.

4. Which personality characteristics would make a person more susceptible to burnout?

    a.   average intelligence, procrastinator, poor health

    b.   above average intelligence, idealistic, perfectionist

    c.   below average intelligence, procrastinator, excellent health

d.   average motivation level, high income, idealistic

5.   Which career characteristics contribute LEAST to the development of burnout?

a.   demand for high quality performance, and unclear expectations

b.   unrealistic expectations, and little control over work situations

c.   high degree of responsibility, and appreciation of work being done.

d.   inadequate financial rewards, and high stress levels.

6.   Which of the following are the most common emotions experienced by nurses who are developing burnout?

a.   Eagerness

b.   Powerlessness

c.   Compassion

d.   Sympathy

7.   The most important characteristic of personal long term goals is that they:

a.   Are planned for at least 10 years in the future

b.   Can be achieved exactly as planned

c.   Remain flexible

d.   Consider every possible contingency along the way

8.	Short term personal goals are goals that the nurse should expect to complete in:

  a.	6 to 24 months

  b.	3 to 4 years

  c.	5 to 10 years

  d.	10 to 20 years

9.	The most important aspect of time management is:

  a.	Doing the job yourself

  b.	Doing the job well no matter how long it takes

  c.	Setting priorities

  d.	Establishing long term goals

10.	Which of the following would be designated Category A tasks that the nurse needs to completed on time?

  a.	Cleaning up the room and combing the client's hair

  b.	Charting and daily bath

  c.	Lunch break and changing the linen

  d.	Giving treatments and changing dressings

11.	In seeking a first job in nursing, the resume:

  a.	Is of little use because most hospitals have a job application form

  b.	Should be as long as possible to impress the interviewer

  c.	Provides the hospital with a complete picture of the graduate in as little space as possible

  d.	Usually has a negative effect on the reader

12. Which of the following individuals should not be listed on the "References" sheet attached to the resume?

   a. The applicant's mother and father

   b. The Dean of the School of Nursing where the applicant graduated

   c. One of the applicant's professors

   d. One of the applicant's fellow students

13. Which of the following questions should the new graduate anticipate being asked during the job interview?

   a. What would make you more desirable as an employee than the other applicants for this job?

   b. Do you attend church regularly and what church to you go to?

   c. Are you planning to become pregnant in the near future?

   d. Are you married to the person you are presently living with?

14. Which question should the new graduate ask first during the interview for a new job?

   a. What is the salary for this position?

   b. What responsibilities are involved in this position?

   c. How much vacation will I get during the first year?

   d. What are my chances for promotion?

Answers

1-c	6-b	11-c
2-d	7-c	12-a
3-a	8-a	13-a
4-b	9-c	14-d
5-c	10-d	

CASE STUDY - THE NURSE AND THE CONTRACT

Betty A, RN, had graduated from an AD program two years ago and was now the 3 to 11 charge nurse on the medical unit of a small rural hospital. Most of her experience for the past two years had been in the medical unit, although she had occasionally floated to the maternity unit, Emergency Room (ER), and Intensive Care Unit (ICU). The usual staffing for her unit on her shift was an RN, an LPN, and an aid.

One Friday evening, the nursing supervisor called Betty at the beginning of her shift and stated that she needed Betty to go to the six bed ICU to cover for 1 to 1.5 hour(s) because the scheduled RN for the ICU had been in a minor accident on the way to work. The supervisor felt Betty was the best qualified of the nurses that were in the hospital at that time, and that the medical unit was quiet enough so that the LPN could handle it while Betty was gone.

Betty quickly went to the ICU where she received an abbreviated report on the four unit patients from the 7 to 3 nurses who were waiting to leave for the weekend. The day shift RN also mentioned that there was a patient in the ER who was experiencing some chest pain and might be admitted to the ICU. Within minutes of receiving report, the ER called and said they were admitting a 46 year old male with an acute anterior myocardial infarction (MI) to the ICU. They also relayed the fact that they had begun streptokinase therapy and the patient would require very close monitoring for dysrhythmias, blood pressure changes, and bleeding.

Betty had never administered or cared for a patient receiving streptokinase and felt incompetent to care for such a patient. Although the LPN working with her had worked with these types of patients, she was not permitted to administer any of the many IV medications this type of patient requires. Just as the patient was being brought through the ICU doors, Betty called the nursing supervisor to let her know that she would need help with this patient. The nursing supervisor said that there was no help available at this time due to call-ins, but that Betty just needed to admit the patient. The regular ICU RN should be in at any time.

Betty assessed the patient and checked his vital signs. He was cold, diaphoretic, and a pale, grey color. His blood pressure was 88/42, pulse of 52, and he was having frequent premature ventricular contractions (PVCs). The monitor tech also informed Betty that he was in a 2:1 AV block. Betty wanted the supervisor to come to the floor and relieve her of the responsibility for the care of this patient. Betty did not know the ICU protocols for dysrhythmia and did not feel competent to care for this seriously ill patient. It would be at least another 45 minutes before the regular RN would arrive.

What are Betty's obligations under her contract with the hospital? What are the hospital's obligations in this situation? Where do the issues of justice and fidelity fit into this situation? Is there any "fidelity conflicts" in this situation? How should Betty resolve the dilemma?

(Aiken, TD, Legal, Ethical, and Political Issues In Nursing FA Davis, Philadelphia 1995.)

Additional Critical Thinking Exercises

1. Have the students identify areas in their lives where they feel they have poor time management. Use the elements in personal time management to resolve these problems.

2. Ask the students to prepare a sample resume and letter to the employer. Working in small groups, have them exchange the resumes and letters and critique them.

3.   Role play an employment interview with a student. Have the other students critique how the interview went and any mistakes the student made.

4.   Have the students bring in the employment advertisement section of a Sunday newspaper. Analyze the adds for nursing positions as to appropriateness for new graduates, qualifications, and any indications of bias.

Chapter 8: Licensure, Certification, Organizations

This chapter begins with a discussion of the purpose of licensure and certification in today's health care system as it evolved over the past 100 years. Distinction is made between the different types of licensure and the implications for health care. Licensure is then related to the nurse practice act and the elements that are found in it. The students are introduced to the concept of certification and how it differs from licensure. The origins of the major nursing organizations are discussed, with current roles, membership requirements, and services offered by the organizations. Special interest organizations in nursing are also presented.

Teaching Points

1. Acquaint the students with the concept, purpose, and nature of licensure in general and in nursing in particular.
2. Discuss the differences and implications of permissive licensure, mandatory licensure, and institutional licensure.
3. Present nurse practice acts, why they are important, and how they affect the practice of the nurse.
4. Differentiate certification from licensure. Discuss the legal and professional implications of certification.
5. Introduce the concept of professional organizations as one of the key elements in a profession. Stress the importance of belonging to a professional organization, and the benefits to the profession and nurses.
6. Describe the two major professional nursing organizations, their functions, membership, and goals. Discuss the Student Nurses Organization and its importance to the nursing student.

7.   List some of the specialty organizations in nursing and describe their function.

Questions

1.   An important element in establishing a nurse support network is to:
      a.   Insist that all nurses follow the same path to success
      b   Avoid criticizing each other in public
      c.   Set very high standards for care
      d.   All of the above

2.   Licensure of nurses was established to:
      a.   Guarantee high quality nurses.
      b.   Increase tax revenues for the state.
      c.   Set a minimum level of competency to protect the public.
      d.   Keep the number in the profession from getting to great.

3   A mandatory nurse practice act is one that requires a nurse to be:
      a.   Employed under the general supervision of a licensed physician
      b.   Currently licensed in the state where the nurse wishes to practice nursing
      c.   Graduated by a school accredited by a national nursing organization
      d.   Enrolled at least yearly in courses approved by the state to meet requirements for continuing education

4.   Which of the following most accurately describes RN licensure in the United States?

   a.   Optional

   b.   Compulsory

   c.   Customary

   d.   Traditional

5.   The main purpose of professional organizations in relationship to a profession is to:

   a.   Collect dues and fund research.

   b.   Monitor practice and discipline incompetent practitioners.

   c.   Fund political actions groups.

   d.   Establish standards for quality practice in the profession.

6.   The listing of names of individuals on an official roster when they have met certain pre-established criteria is called:

   a.   Certification

   b.   Licensure

   c.   Registration

   d.   All of the above

7.   Permissive licensure:

   a.   Only protects the title "Registered Nurse"

   b.   Allows anyone to use the title "Registered Nurse"

   c.   As found in most states

   d.   Can be used by institutions when hiring foreign nurses

8. The most serious problem with institutional licensure is:

   a. The standards are too difficult for most nurses to meet.

   b. It makes moving from one institution to another more difficult.

   c. Many qualified individuals would be excluded from the profession.

   d. There are no external controls to determine a minimum level of ability.

9. A type of credentialing that indicates that an individual has achieved a high level of expertise and knowledge in an area of practice is called:

   a. Licensure

   b. Certification

   c. Professionalism

   d. Registration

10. The primary purpose of the National League for Nursing is to:

    a. Establish standards of practice to insure high quality care.

    b. Maintain and improve the standards of nursing education.

    c. Increase the political power of nurses to influence legislation.

    d. Prevent unqualified nurses from practicing in hospitals.

11. Which of the following is NOT one of the goals of the American Nurses Association?

    a. Maintain and improve the standards of nursing education.

    b. Promotion of the professional growth and development of all nurses.

    c. Improve the access to health care services for everyone.

    d. Increasing the independence of practice by nurses.

12. The primary membership in the American Nurses Association is:

   a. Schools of nursing

   b. Health care facilities such as hospitals

   c. Individual nurses

   d. State nursing organizations

13. Which of the following is NOT a service provided by the ANA?

   a. Testing and certification of advanced practice nurses

   b. Establishing entry level requirements for nurses

   c. Updating the standards of nursing practice

   d. Accreditation of schools of nursing

14. The National Student Nurses Organization has as its primary purpose:

   a. Changing curriculums in schools of nursing to allow more students to pass.

   b. Eliminating poor and unprofessional nursing professors from schools of nursing.

   c. Maintaining high standards of education in schools of nursing.

   d. Keeping unqualified students from entering the profession.

15. What is the most significant benefit to a student who belongs to the National Student Nurses Association?

   a. Receiving the official publication, **_IMPRINT_**, along with the membership.

   b. Experiencing first hand the operation, activities, and professionalism of a national organization.

   c. Obtaining one of the many large cash scholarships available through the organization.

d.   Joining an elite group who have a great deal of power and a
       wide range of control over other students.

Answers

1-b	6-c	11-a
2-c	7-a	12-c
3-b	8-d	13-d
4-b	9-b	14-c
5-d	10-b	15-b

Additional Critical Thinking Exercises

1.   Name the key elements found in licensure laws.
2.   Analyze the development and importance of the licensure
       examination.
3.   List the main reasons why a nursing license may be revoked.
4.   Prepare a presentation for a group of new graduate nurses entitled
       "Why I should belong to the ANA."
5.   Develop a description of a health care system where nurses are not
       required to be licensed.
6.   Identify threats to current nursing practice from unlicensed personnel,
       and propose solutions to this trend.
10.   Outline a method for organizing a central agency for all nurse
       certifications, including location, organizational chart, and governing
       body. What would be the best way to implement this plan in the
       shortest amount of time?

Additional Student Activities

Match the term, organization, or abbreviation from column B with the appropriate answer in column A.

Column A	Column B
_____ The professional organization for registered nurses located in Washington DC.	1. American Nurse
_____ The initials after a nurse's name designating passing of the licensing exam.	2. Imprint
_____ The official journal of the ANA.	3. Code of Ethics
_____ Nursing organization concerned primarily with educational standards of nursing schools.	4. Registration
_____ Document first published in 1950 that serves as a guide for ethical nursing practice.	5. ANA
_____ The listing of individuals who have met established criteria.	6. NLN
_____ Individuals who provide low level health care who are not licensed.	7. RN
_____ A type of advanced certification for nurses who provide care to children.	8. PNP
_____ The official publication of the NSNA.	9. UAP

Order of Answers: 5,7,1,6,3,4,9,8,2

Chapter 9: NCLEX - What Students Need to Know

Chapter 9 acquaints the student with purpose and format of the NCLEX examination. The major components of the NCLEX-RN, CAT (Nursing Process, Client Health Needs, Levels of Cognitive Ability) are discussed and explained with examples of the various type of questions that may be found in each component. The examination format is explored, including the type of questions used, the "grading system" for the examination, and the maximum and minimum number of questions required. An example is presented of a question on a computer screen. Several different study strategies are presented to the student for use when studying for the NCLEX or any type of multiple choice examination. The chapter ends with a presentation of selected test taking strategies that may help the student improve his or her grade on this type of test.

Teaching Points

1.   Review the nursing process and demonstrate how it is used in questions on the NCLEX examination.

2.   Discuss the four Client Health Needs categories, including the major content included in each area. Give examples of a question from each area.

3.   Analyze the idea of levels of cognitive ability. Stress the fact that the majority of the questions on the NCLEX are at the higher levels.

4.   Describe the NCLEX examinations computer format, how a passing score is reached, and the physical arrangement of the room where the examination is taken.

5.   Present the relative importance of various study strategies such as review books, group study, individual study, and review courses.

6. Review key test taking strategies, using examples wherever possible.

Questions

1. The NCLEX-CAT, RN is:

   a. A certification examination taken by all nurses

   b. Too difficult for most new graduates to pass the first time

   c. Unnecessary in states where institutional licensure is the rule

   d. Required by all nurses for licensure

2. For the NCLEX-CAT, RN, the nursing process is:

   a. A five step process involving assessment, analysis, planning, implementation, and evaluation

   b. A four step process involving assessment, planning, implementation, and evaluation

   c. Unimportant and no questions are asked about it

   d. The most important part of the examination

3. Which of the following stem questions would best indicate that an "Evaluation" category question was being asked?

   a. Which of the following actions should the nurse perform first?

   b. You would know your teaching concerning colostomy care was successful if the client states?

   c. Which of the following data is most important to obtain on a client with cardiac disease?

   d. Of the following four nursing diagnosis, which one has the highest priority?

4.   Which of the following stem questions would best indicate that an
        "Assessment" category question was being asked?
        a.   Which of the following actions should the nurse perform first?
        b.   You would know your teaching concerning colostomy care
                was successful if the client states?
        c.   Which of the following data is most important to obtain on a
                client with cardiac disease?
        d.   Of the following four nursing diagnosis, which one has the
                highest priority?

5.   Which of the following stem questions would best indicate that an
        "Analysis" category question was being asked?
        a.   Which of the following actions should the nurse perform first?
        b.   You would know your teaching concerning colostomy care
                was successful if the client states?
        c.   Which of the following data is most important to obtain on a
                client with cardiac disease?
        d.   Of the following four nursing diagnosis, which one has the
                highest priority?

6.   Which of the following stem questions would best indicate that an
        "Implementation" category question was being asked?
        a.   Which of the following actions should the nurse perform first?
        b.   You would know your teaching concerning colostomy care
                was successful if the client states?
        c.   Which of the following data is most important to obtain on a
                client with cardiac disease?
        d.   Of the following four nursing diagnosis, which one has the
                highest priority?

7. In which of the following health needs categories of the NCLEX-CAT, RN examination would the student find questions about a pregnant woman?

    a. Safe and effective care environment

    b. Psychosocial needs

    c. Health promotion and maintenance needs

    d. Physiological needs

8. A stem questions states: "A client admitted with BUN of 64, and a Creatinine of 6 would require which of the following nursing actions first?" What cognitive level does this stem question indicate?

    a. Level 1, recall question

    b. Level 2, analysis question

    c. Level 3, synthesis question

    d. Level 4, advanced question

9. The maximum number of questions that a graduate may answer on the NCLEX-RN CAT is:

    a. 75

    b. 265

    c. 370

    d. 500

10. In the abbreviation, NCLEX-CAT, RN, the CAT stands for:

    a. Computerized assistive testing

    b. Complex assessment technique

    c. Computerized assessment testing

    d. Computerized adaptive testing

11. Which of the following is true about the NCLEX-CAT, RN?

    a. Partial credit is given for close answers.

    b. The examination is given at the Silvan Learning Centers.

    c. High levels of computer skills are needed to complete the test successfully.

    d. The graduate is allowed to go back and change the answers of questions answered previously on the exam.

12. A graduate who fails the NCLEX-CAT, RN:

    a. must wait at least 45 days before retaking it

    b. only has to retake the portion of the exam that was failed

    c. can never become a registered nurse

    d. can retake the examination immediately

13. Graduates who decide to use group study as a means of preparing for the NCLEX-CAT, RN, should:

    a. Get a group of at least 15 students for optimal study.

    b. Make sure that study sessions are at least 3 hours long for the most efficient use of time.

    c. Have each group member prepare a section of the topic for study during that session.

    d. Bring chips, candy, pizza and soda to the session to maintain the energy levels.

14. When taking a multiple choice examination such as the NCLEX-CAT, RN, it is important to:

 a. Read each question over and over so that related information can be remembered.

 b. Select the first answer that is correct to save time.

 c. Ignore negative words in the stem question because they confuse the issue.

 d. Trust intuition and avoid reading into the question.

15. Which of the following words in a stem question would make the question negative?

 a. First

 b. Atypical

 c. Highest Priority

 d. Appropriate

Answers

1-d	6-a	11-b
2-a	7-c	12-a
3-b	8-c	13-c
4-c	9-b	14-d
5-d	10-d	15-b

Additional Critical Thinking Exercises

1. Have the students write 10 sample NCLEX examination questions from content they are covering in their current courses.

2. In conjunction with the students, rank the questions on the next examination as to level of difficulty (1 to 6).

3. Obtain and install a sample NCLEX-RN, CAT on a computer and have the students take the examination.

4. Have the student identify the category of health care need indicated by each of the following questions. Discuss why they are in that category.

(Key: 1 = Physiological needs; 2 = Psychosocial needs; 3 = Health promotion and maintenance; 4 = Safe and effective care environment

QUESTION	1	2	3	4
A 38 year old client is 15 weeks pregnant. What should the nurse teach her about weight gain?				
What would be the most appropriate goal for a client admitted with abdominal pain, vomiting, and bloody stools?				
Of the following four toys, which one would be most appropriate for an 8 month old?				
Which of the following is the most important information to obtain on a client who overdosed on amphetamines?				
What would be an appropriate nursing measure for a client admitted to the hospital who has a potassium of 6.3?				
Which of the following would be the best response by the nurse to a client with a myocardial infarction who asks if he is dying?				
Which complications should the nurse monitor a client for who is to have a paracervical block?				
Which measures would reduce a client's discomfort from dumping syndrome?				
A nurse notices that a coworker has a strong smell of alcohol on her breath at the beginning of the shift. What would be the most appropriate action by the nurse at this time?				
While bathing a client with chest tubes, the notices bubbling in the waterseal chamber. This most likely indicates:				

Chapter 10: Health Care Delivery

Beginning with a brief historical review of the health care system in the United States, Chapter 10 defines key terms used in describing health care delivery, discusses the prime members of the health care time, and presents the main factors that influence current health care delivery practices. Because monetary concerns are an integral part of current health care reform proposals, payment systems for health care are explored in depth. Common elements of the many proposed health care reforms are discussed, with a presentation of managed care systems in the context of their original design. The concept of quality assurance is introduced. The final part of the chapter presents the current methods of health care delivery.

Teaching Points

1. Explain how the current health care system in the United States evolved from earlier forms of health care delivery. Point out why past delivery systems do not work today, including factors found in modern health care that were not present in the past.

2. Define key terms used in health care delivery such as primary, secondary, and tertiary care, and discuss the key health care providers.

3. Analyze why there are rising costs in health care and explain the pros and cons of the various systems for payment.

4. Discuss current health care industry attempts to control health care costs including managed care, independent practice associations, preferred provider organizations, and group practice arrangements. What are the strong and weak points of each of these systems?

5. Define quality assurance. Why has it become so important in today's health care system? How does it affect nurses?

6.   Define and describe the various forms of health care delivery
      currently being used. Which are most effective? What are the
      limitations of the various forms of delivery?

Questions

1.   Acute care of the sick that is provided in the hospital is called:
      a.   Primary intervention
      b.   Secondary intervention
      c.   Tertiary intervention
      d.   Assistive intervention

2.   One negative result of the centralization of health care in hospitals
      rather than the home setting was:
      a.   Individual responsibility was minimized
      b.   Increased concerns about the cost of health care
      c.   Professionalization of nursing
      d.   Increased reliance on advanced technology

3.   The current trend towards decentralized health care includes all of the
      following except:
      a.   Provision of care on an outpatient basis
      b.   Emphasis on cure of illness
      c.   Promotion of responsible self-care practices
      d.   Cost containment measures by health care providers

4.   Which demographic factor has the most significant effect upon the
      health care delivery system of the future?
      a.   The large numbers of babies being born to minority women

b. The increasing use of alcohol and tobacco among teenagers

c. The rapidly increasing average age of the population

d. The oversupply of nurses.

5. Health care costs continue to rise in the United States due to:

a. Expensive new technology

b. Increasing need for long term care

c. Lack of motivation for consumers to comparison shop

d. All of the above

6. The most important reason why nurses should be familiar with health care reimbursement methods is because:

a. It allows nurses to be informed client advocates

b. Nursing care plans can be developed based upon financial incentives to lower costs

c. Nurses can decide which tests do and do not need to be conducted on clients

d. Decisions can be made about when a client can be discharged based on reimbursement restrictions

7. One of the major difficulties with self-insured health care plans is:

a. Increased cost to the members

b. Shielding from many state tax regulations

c. Exclusion of potential employees based on past health history

d. Elimination of outside regulators to supervise private insurance plans

8. Which of the following is a result of past difficulties with the Blue Cross or Blue Shield insurance plans?

    a. Increased emphasis on preventative health care

    b. Involvement of the hospital boards of directors to lower costs

    c. More private insurance companies administering Blue Cross or Blue Shield programs

    d. Transfer of more power to physicians' groups to monitor the flow of money within the program

9. Diagnosis related groups (DRGs) is the primary form of:

    a. Private insurance companies

    b. Prospective payment systems

    c. Retrospective payment systems

    d. Current reimbursement systems

10. Which methods are used by HMOs to reduce the cost of health care delivery?

    a. Increasing the number of diagnostic studies to detect diseases early

    b. Encouraging clients to remain in the hospital longer so that they can recover completely and not be readmitted

    c. Referring more clients to specialists so that complex health care problems can be treated better

    d. Providing more health promotion and illness prevention services

11. The primary difference between HMOs and Independent Practice Associations (IPAs) is that under the IPA system:
    a. Physicians loose much of their control over health care delivery.
    b. Clients pay on fee-for-service basis rather than prepaid premiums.
    c. Nurses receive reimbursement for the care they provide on an individual basis.
    d. The number of services provided is not limited.

12. The major advantage that Preferred Provider Organization (PPO) payment systems have over HMO is that the PPO:
    a. Extends benefits beyond the use of their services at an increased rate
    b. Plan requires co-payment fees each time a service is rendered
    c. Services are used by a smaller number of clients thus reducing the wait for services
    d. System reduces costs more

13. The key element in the horizontal integration of health care services is:
    a. The use of a fee-for-service method of payment.
    b. One hospital providing the entire scope of services so that client's can be cared for without referral outside the system.
    c. Several health care agencies working together to cut costs by sharing resources.
    d. The development of clinics outside the hospital to provide services traditionally found in the hospital.

14. Nurse run clinics have as their primary focus:

    a. Health promotion

    b. Disease prevention

    c. Counseling services

    d. All of the above

15. Which of the following factors is most important in the increased development of alternative ambulatory services?

    a. Increased length of hospital stays

    b. New technology made complicated and dangerous procedures available on an outpatient basis

    c. Consumer demand for more technology in the cure of disease

    d. The establishment of satellite clinics in suburbs and rural communities

Answers

1-b	6-a	11-b
2-a	7-c	12-a
3-b	8-c	13-c
4-c	9-b	14-d
5-d	10-d	15-b

CASE STUDY - CHANGING A CHART

It was an extremely busy 3 to 11 shift on the surgical unit of a large city hospital. Because it was a Wednesday evening, the unit was not only receiving fresh postoperative patients from surgery, but was also in the process of discharging patients and admitting new patients for the next day's surgery schedule.

Melinda L, RN, charge nurse for the 3 to 11 shift, had worked on the surgical unit for two years. She had a reputation for being a well organized, competent, and hard-working nurse who seemed to be able to bring order out of chaos. On this particular, even her considerable skills in organization were failing to settle the unit to a point where she felt in control.

Mrs. Star J, an 66 year old diabetic, was being admitted at 4:00 pm to the surgical unit because of poor circulation in her legs and possible infection of her right foot. One of her admission orders was to culture the drainage from the sore on her great right toe. In checking the orders after the unit secretary had noted them, Melinda decided to do the culture herself because all of her staff was already tied up in other activities. Melinda explained the procedure to Mrs. J, and then proceeded to culture a draining sore on her left toe. The culture was taken to the lab with the appropriate slips by the unit secretary.

During supper that evening, a patient aspirated and coded. A little later, a patient fell while attempting to climb out of bed with the bed rails up. It was almost 11:45 pm when Melinda finally got to sit down and do her charting. After all that had happened that evening, she was having some trouble remembering what she had done earlier in the shift.

When she came to Mrs. J's chart, she remembered that she had gotten a culture, and checked back on the orders to make sure it was actually ordered. The order said "C&S right great toe" so Melinda charted, "1630 -

Culture of right great toe obtained and sent to lab. Procedure explained to patient." and signed it.

On her way home that night, Melinda was thinking about how busy the shift was and all that had happened. She wondered if she had done everything that was supposed to be done, and charted everything that needed to be charted. She also began thinking about Mrs. J and the culture. By the time she reached home, she felt pretty sure that she had cultured the wrong toe. She would correct the chart in two days when she worked again.

When Melinda returned after her two days off, she discovered that Mrs. J had a below the knee amputation of her right leg. The physician had decided to do the amputation because the culture that was sent to the lab had grown *Clostridium perfringens* (gas gangrene). Melinda feels that she is responsible for this mistake. What should she do? If she "tells" or tries to correct the chart, she could be open to a law suit.

(Aiken, TD: <u>Legal, Ethical, and Political Issues In Nursing</u> FA Davis, Philadelphia 1995.)

Additional Critical Thinking Exercises

1. Propose three new roles for nurses within the future revised health care delivery system in the United States.
2. Discuss the benefits of group practice arrangements. How can nurses become involved in these practices?
3. Visit a home health care agency and a public health department in your community. How are these similar and how do they differ? Include funding for services, type of client, and staffing.
4. Analyze how the power structure of health care might change as health care delivery is modernized. Who has the most power in the

current system? Who stands to lose power and who will gain power? How do nurses fare in these changes?

Chapter 11: Politically Active Nurse

In Chapter 11, the student is introduced to the political process in general, and its effect on health care in particular. The chapter begins with a presentation of current political action and how it affects health care. The various levels of political activity are discussed and examples are given of involvement of nurses at each level. The structure and function of government is outlined, with a discussion of how and where laws are made. A model for political activism is discussed including the various levels of involvement (civic, advocacy, organization, and long-term). Why and how to communicate with legislators is presented and a discussion of the political significance of professional organizations is emphasized. The chapter concludes with a presentation on political action committees and political nursing network and coalitions.

Teaching Points

1. Discuss why it is essential that nurses become involved in politics at some level in today's health care system.
2. Describe the levels of political involvement possible by nurses and give examples of how nurses can become active at the levels.
3. Outline the structure and function of government, including the three branches.
4. Describe how a law is made, and best points in the process to make changes in the law.
5. List and define the activities for becoming more involved in the political process.

6. Identify the best means for communicating with legislators. Stress the importance of professional organization membership as a form of political power.

7. Define and explain political action committees and political nursing networks and coalitions. Why are these important?

Questions

1. The act or science of influencing public policy best describes:
    a.   Power
    b.   Nursing
    c.   Politics
    d.   Ethics

2. The document that provides nurses with the right to practice and specifies the parameters of professional practice is called:
    a.   Nurse Practice Act
    b.   Scope of Practice
    c.   Legislative Law
    d.   State Board of Nursing

3. Decisions that are made by the State Board of Nursing:
    a.   Influence all aspects of the health care system
    b.   Have the same force as law
    c.   Are recommendations that may or may not be followed
    d.   Must be approved by a majority of nurses in the state

4.   The sphere of political influence where optimum working conditions are created and quality client care is assured is the:

a.   Community

b.   Government

c.   Workplace

d.   Organization

5.   Which of the following would be the best method for nurses to influence those in power?

a.   Taking an active role in institutional decisions making

b.   Remaining current with trends and issues in nursing

c.   Serving on hospital and community health care committees

d.   All of the above

6.   Which of the following would be appropriate political activities for nurses at the state level?

a.   Introduce legislation and seek sponsors.

b.   Vote in the legislature for or against a bill.

c.   Make large monetary contributions to candidates who support health reform.

d.   Keep quiet and let the system work without interference.

7.   The most important reason that the input of nurses is vital to legislators is because:

a.   Most of the bills legislators pass are not related to health care.

b.   Voters can be easily misled by special interest groups.

c.   The majority of legislator do not have a health care background.

d.   Legislators need to be aware of the important part nurses play in the health care system.

8.   The best way for nurses to influence the legislative process at the federal level is to:

    a.   Organize demonstrations outside the White House when important health care issues are discussed.

    b.   Send telegrams and letters to their congressman and representatives in the house.

    c.   Have the main nursing organizations speak with a unified voice when presenting their concerns.

    d.   Join and actively participate in hospital committees on health care.

9.   A Board of Supervisors is usually found in which type of government structure?

    a.   State

    b.   County

    c.   Federal

    d.   City

10.   Which of the following comprise the branches found in the government at the federal level?

    a.   Legislative, executive

    b.   Executive, judicial, president

    c.   Congress, legislative, judicial

    d.   Legislative, executive, judicial

11. Which of the following Congressional committees is responsible for dealing with health legislation in general?

    a. Senate Finance Committee

    b. Senate Labor and Human Resources Committee

    c. House Commerce Committee

    d. House Ways and Means Committee

12. The primary responsibility of the Rules Committee is to:

    a. Schedule bills and determine how much time will be spent on debate.

    b. Oversee the whole legislative process to prevent errors in a bill's development.

    c. Decide whether a bill may be reported out favorably or killed.

    d. Establish the guidelines for the progression of the bill through a committee.

13. If the House and Senate have different version of the same bill, the bills then goes to the:

    a. President for signature of the bill he favors most

    b. Rules Committee to set up the guidelines for passage of the bill

    c. Conference Committee to resolve the differences between the two bills

    d. Finance Committee to see if there is enough money in the budget for both forms

14. Which of the following are valuable sources of information about political issues that affect the profession of nursing?

    a. *The American Nurse*

    b. *Nursing and Health Care*

    c. *Capitol Update*

    d. All of the above

15. The primary purpose of the American Nurses Association-Political Action Committees

    (ANA-PACs) is to:

    a. Persuade public officials to work for legislation nurses consider important.

    b. Influence the outcome of elections.

    c. Prevent bills that are negative for nursing from being introduced in Congress.

    d. Attempt to change the minds of Legislators already serving in Congress.

Answers

1-c	6-a	11-b
2-a	7-c	12-a
3-b	8-c	13-c
4-c	9-b	14-d
5-d	10-d	15-b

Additional Critical Thinking Exercises

1. Have the students contact the state board of nursing of their state, and
    see if there is a functioning political action committee in the state.
    Contact the PAC and find out what issues it is promoting.

2. Divide the class into small groups. Have each group select a political
    issue they feel strongly about. Have the group identify 2 to 3
    legislators that may influence the issue and write letters to these
    individuals supporting or opposing the selected issue. Report the
    results to the class.

3. Divide the class in half. Have one half present a position on support
    of health care reform, and the other half against reform. What are the
    rationales? What are the consequences of their positions?

4. Give the students a list of the current health care related issues before
    Congress. Have them rank them from highest to lowest priority.
    Analyze why the positions were taken.

Chapter 12: Collective Bargaining and Governance

This chapter begins with a definition and discussion of collective bargaining and its relationship to professional nursing. The history of collective bargaining in the United States is outlined and the goals of collective bargaining are presented. The concerns professional nurses may have about collective bargaining are presented and discussed. The concept of the contract is introduced, and the collective bargaining process is outlined. Emphasis is placed on representation for collective bargaining, with the advantages and disadvantages of SNA and unions being discussed. The implications of 1994 Supreme Court decision concerning collective bargaining is presented. The chapter concludes with a discussion of governance, the roles of nurses in governance, and several different models for governance.

Teaching Points

1. Define collective bargaining, present its goals and purposes, and explain its evolution.
2. List the primary concerns professional nurses have about collective bargaining. Discuss each concern.
3. Outline the collective bargaining process and discuss the contract as the goal. What elements are important in a good contract?
4. Discuss the Taft-Hartley Act and relate the 1994 Supreme Court decision to this act. Analyze its affect on current collective bargaining attempts by RNs.
5. Define governance. Explain how nurses are affected by governance.
6. Present and analyze various models for governance as to their implications for professional nurses.

Questions

1. What is the most likely reason that nurses have traditionally avoid joining unions and participating in collective bargaining?
   a. The unions had little to offer nurses as far as pay and working conditions were concerned.
   b. Unions were largely male dominated organizations and wanted little to do with nursing.
   c. Joining a union seemed to contradict nursing's image of dedication, service, and selflessness.
   d. Nurses already had a great deal of control over their working conditions, salaries, or benefits.

2. Collective bargaining is best defined as:
   a. A conflict-based power strategy used to equalize the power between labor and management
   b. The right of all workers to organize and strike to gain more benefits
   c. The ability of large numbers of workers to force management into recognizing them as valuable
   d. Using picket lines, and violence to achieve higher pay, better working conditions, and shorter hours

3. A law that was passed in 1935 that allowed employees the right to self-organization and formation of unions for the purpose of collective bargaining is called:
   a. American Labor Union Act
   b. National Labor Relations Act

c.   Employees Self-Determination Act

d.   Right-To-Strike Law

4.   An important consequence of the Supreme Court ruling in 1991 concerning collective bargaining units for health care providers was that it:

a.   Eliminated the right of nurses and other health care providers to join unions

b.   Excluded non-profit hospitals and their employees from coverage by the National Labor Relations Board

c.   Permitted all RN bargaining units to be formed

d.   Defined ten separate bargaining units that were appropriate for hospitals

5.   In relationship to collective bargaining, the American Nurses Association (ANA):

a.   Is the primary bargaining unit for nurses across the country

b.   Is opposed to collective bargaining by nurses because it is unprofessional

c.   Recommends that nurses join powerful unions such as the AFL-CIO to maximize their power

d.   Actively supports the State Nurses Associations (SNAs) to function as bargaining agents

6.   Which of the following is the most accurate statement about the power that employees have in an organization?

a.   Employees have more power than they realize because the organization is dependent on them to carry out its goals.

b. Employees have very little power in any organization because they are located at the bottom of power structure hierarchy.

c. Individual employees can have a significant effect on management when they initiate change in the work setting.

d. Management has the ultimate power over employees because it is easy to replace unhappy employees with other individuals from the large pool of unemployed.

7. A goal of collective bargaining that is often overlooked by management but is important to nursing is:

a. Improved staffing, and higher quality personnel

b. Better salaries, and more benefits

c. Maintaining and promoting professional practice

d. Overtime pay, and personal holidays

8. In attempting to decide whether or not to go on strike, nurses are often concerned about the wellbeing of the clients in the hospital. Which of the following legal requirements helps alleviate this concern?

a. Hospitals are permitted to hire unlicensed personnel to substitute for the striking RNs.

b. Enough RNs are required to stay and work on the floors to maintain safe levels of care.

c. A 10 day notice must be given to the hospital before a strike takes place.

d. LPNs are permitted to function as RNs in a strike situation.

9.   Important factors in the initial negotiation of a contract include:

    a.   Discussion of the important issues

    b.   Posturing and showmanship

    c.   Resolution of key conflicts

    d.   Lack of willingness to negotiate

10.   Which of the following are usually considered to be unfair labor practices?

    a.   Being fired because a physician does not like a nurse's attitude

    b.   Being passed over for promotion without being given any explanation

    c.   Being assigned to work five weekends in a row when the policy is every other weekend off

    d.   All of the above

11.   Which of the following would be an indication of failure to bargain in good faith?

    a.   Agreeing to meet at reasonable times

    b.   Sending individuals to negotiate who can not make binding decisions

    c.   Unwillingness to negotiate on all issues

    d.   Exchanging a list of demands by both sides.

12.   The primary role of the Federal Mediation and Conciliation Service is to:

    a.   Bring both sides together to work out a settlement

    b.   Prevent nurses, and other health care groups from going on strike

    c.   Develop a solution to the conflict that is binding on both sides

d.   Force management into accepting the employee demands

13.   What is the most important advantage that a union has over a SNA as a bargaining unit for nurses?

a.   The union has a good understanding of the complex needs of the profession.

b.   The union has more power as a bargaining unit than an SNA.

c.   Unions have skilled representatives with much experience in negotiating contracts.

d.   Hospitals and nursing homes are more afraid of unions than SNAs.

14.   Which of the following would be important elements to look for in a good contract?

a.   Description of the official bargaining group

b.   Description of the benefits included in the contract such as wages, overtime pay, holidays, and so on

c.   Description of what is expected of the professional

d.   All of the above

15.   The most important feature of the shared governance model is:

a.   Nursing administration retains most of the power over nurses to better regulate practice.

b.   Power and authority is transferred to the nursing staff rather than being located primarily in nursing administration.

c.   Clients are billed for nursing care as a separate item similar to the way they are billed for physician services.

d.   The nursing staff hierarchy structure is similar to the medical staff structure.

Answers

1-c	6-a	11-b
2-a	7-c	12-a
3-b	8-c	13-c
4-c	9-b	14-d
5-d	10-d	15-b

CASE STUDY - MAKING A FATAL MEDICATION ERROR

David B, 56 years old, was admitted to the intensive care unit (ICU) with severe chest pain and a diagnosis of an acute anterior myocardial infarction (MI). After several hours in the unit, he began to have short runs (5 to 10 beats) of ventricular tachycardia (VT) that ended without treatment. The physician was called and an order for lidocaine was obtained.

Karen M, who was Mr. B's nurse, took the phone order for the medication. In writing down the order, she mistakenly wrote "1000 mg IV bolus, followed by a drip at 2 mg per minute," rather than "100 mg IV bolus, followed by drip at 2 mg per minute." Amanda K, another RN who had been pulled to the ICU from the pediatric unit offered to give the medication because Karen was so busy. Amanda gave the medication as the order was written and Mr. B promptly went into cardiac arrest. Resuscitative measures including a pacemaker proved futile in reviving him.

It was only after the code was over, and Karen was completing her chart that she realized her error in writing down a dose that was 10 times more than what was the usual dose. If she had been giving the medication herself, she would have discovered the error immediately, but the pediatric nurse was unfamiliar with the ICU medications and had given the full dose. The patient had arrested so quickly after the medication was given that Amanda did not have time to chart it. Because Karen was the only one who has seen the chart and the order, it would be very easy for her to change it. Amanda had already gone back to the pediatric unit and did not even realize she had given a wrong dosage of this lethal medication. It is also likely that no one else would ever discover what really happened to Mr. B.

About that time, Mr. B's wife arrived to collect his personal belongings. She stopped at the desk where Karen was completing her chart to thank Karen for her care of her husband. Karen feels very guilty about the incident, and wonders if she should tell Mr. B's wife what really happened.

What should Karen do? What would be the consequences of the possible choices of action? What ethical principle(s) should underlay Karen's decision?

(Aiken, TD: Legal, Ethical, and Political Issues In Nursing FA Davis, Philadelphia 1995.)

Additional Critical Thinking Exercises

1.   Why does the role of nursing supervisor present problems for nurses when they attempt collective bargaining? Are there any ways that these problems can be overcome?

2.   Plan a strike for the nurses at a facility you are familiar with. Make a list of the problems that may occur as a result of the strike and devise solutions for these problems.

3.   Contact the head of the State Nurses Association and ask if they conduct collective bargaining. If they do not, ask them what would be required to initiate the process in the state.

4.   List alternatives to collective bargaining. What are the benefits and difficulties with these alternatives? Are they as effective as collective bargaining?

Chapter 13: Nursing, Law, and Liability

Chapter 13 introduces the student to the legal world, its terminology, and how law relates to health care and nursing practice. An initial discussion of statutory and common law as the two primary sources for law introduces the chapter. Civil and criminal law are then presented, with an extended discussion of the classifications of violations of civil law (torts). Examples of the various types of torts nurses are most likely to become involved with are included. Self-determination and informed consent are presented as legal concepts and related to DNR orders. Standards of care, and the nurse practice act are presented as the legal standards that nurses are held to. The legal process in a lawsuit is outlined, including the concepts of assumption of risk, Good Samaritan Statues, and unavoidable accidents. Guidelines nurses can use to prevent law suits are discussed.

Teaching Points

1. Discuss the importance of understanding the legal system and the relationship of law to nursing.
2. Outline and define the various types of law (statutory, common, criminal, and civil).
3. Explain the three types of torts and give examples of each type as it relates to a health care incident.
4. Define informed consent and self-determination from a legal standpoint. Discuss the exceptions to these principles and their relationship to DNR orders.
5. Identify standards of care and stress how and why they are important in the legal aspects of nursing.

6. Take the student through the legal process involved in a law suit. Define the terms statute of limitation, answer, complaint, defendant, plaintiff, and discovery.

7. Discuss possible defenses to a malpractice suit.

8. List and discuss ways that nurses can prevent law suits.

9. Discuss the circumstances under which a nursing license might be revoked.

Questions

1. If a patient is not allowed to leave the hospital after receiving emergency care until her bill is paid, the hospital's action can constitute the offense known as:

    a. Assault

    b. Battery

    c. Invasion of privacy

    d. False imprisonment

2. If a nurse tells several friends and coworkers that a patient, who is a physician, is unsafe for medical practice because he is paralyzed from the waist down and acts "slightly silly," the nurse's action can constitute the offense known as:

    a. Libel

    b. Fraud

    c. Slander

    d. Malpractice

3   If the nurse is sued for negligence following the administration of an injection, which one of the following persons will most likely be asked to serve as an expert witness to describe standards of care?

a.   An experienced nursing supervisor or instructor

b.   A lawyer who has successfully defended another nurse sued for negligence

c.   A judge who is considered to be an expert in the field of professional negligence

d.   Another patient who had received an injection by the same nurse but without complications

4.   The nurse working in an emergency room is of the opinion that to carry out a certain order written by a physician could possibly constitute unethical or illegal behavior. Which one of the following courses of action would be best for the nurse to take in this situation?

a.   Carry out the order; then discuss it with the physician.

b.   Carry out the order; then discuss it with your supervisor.

c.   Do not carry out the order; report the situation to the physician.

d.   Do not carry out the order; report the situation to the supervisor.

5.   The best definition of assault is:

a.   Application of force to another person without lawful justification

b.   Threats to do bodily harm to the person of another person

c.   A legal wrong committed by one person against the property of another

d.   A legal wrong committed against the public and punishable by law

6.   Legally, the term *battery* means:

     a.   Doing something that a reasonable person with the same education or preparation would not do

     b.   A legal wrong committed by one person against the property of another

     c.   Application of force to the person of another person without lawful justification or permission

     d.   Maligning the character of an individual while threatening to do bodily harm

7.   Nursing licensure laws are types of:

     a.   Criminal laws

     b.   Contract laws

     c.   Federal laws

     d.   Civil laws

8.   The client's chart is considered to be a legal document and of vital importance in the care of the client. All of the following statements are important facts that should be charted, EXCEPT:

     a.   If the client does not keep follow-up appointments

     b.   If the client discontinues treatment

     c.   If the client refuses medication

     d.   If the nurse thinks the client is hostile.

9. In which of the following situations would an emergency room nurse be justified in proceeding without obtaining consent, verbal, or otherwise?

    a.   An unconscious, profusely bleeding victim is brought in by ambulance

    b.   A 13 year-old child is brought to the ER after suffering a fractured arm while at school

    c.   A construction worker comes into the ER to have a boil lanced

    d.   A 15 year-old high school girl comes in for treatment of psoriasis

10. The right to privacy is a very important right. In which of the following situations is the nurse allowed to violate this right?

    a.   A local politician is admitted after an automobile accident in which he was inebriated

    b.   A 18 year old unwed teenager seeks an abortion at an abortion clinic

    c.   A 32 year old housewife comes to the ER for care after being raped in a parking lot

    d.   An important member of the business community is treated for cuts, and bruises after a fight with his neighbor

11. An 18 month old child is brought into the emergency room with several recent cigarette burns on his chest and legs. He cannot use his left arm, which is edematous. The nurse's legal responsibility in this case is to:

   a. Do nothing immediately, but plan to check the child carefully if it occurs again.

   b. Notify the attending physician and/or the Emergency Room Supervisor.

   c. Tell the mother that he/she suspects abuse and chastise her about her actions.

   d. Since you only have suspicions, remember that an individual is innocent until proven guilty.

12. The newborn nursery is desperately short of staff. The nurse agrees to work an extra shift. During the 14th hour on duty, the nurse makes a medication error. Since the nurse was filling a "desperate" staffing need, and was therefore fatigued:

   a. The hospital accepts the responsibility for the negligent act.

   b. The nurse is held to the same standard of care as any nurse with her education and experience.

   c. No problem exists if the client does not bring legal action.

   d. Legal responsibilities are met if an incident report is filed.

13. Which of the following statements is most accurate in the description of a *Tort*?

   a. It is a violation of the criminal law.

   b. If proven guilty, the defendant will go to prison

   c. It is a violation of the civil law.

   d. It is something that is good to have for breakfast.

14. Which of the following statements is false about a *Tort*?

    a.   If the plaintiff wins, he will be awarded money.

    b.   Intentional torts can sometimes be considered crimes.

    c.   It is considered to be a violation of a personal right.

    d.   It is considered to be a legal wrong against the public.

15. Mr. Smith, a former client of the hospital, alleges that a surgical instrument was left inside his abdominal cavity following surgery. If his allegation is proven to be true, which of the following would be liable in this suit?

    a.   The physician

    b.   The hospital

    c.   The circulating surgical nurse

    d.   All of the above

16. Which of the following is an accurate statement in regards to nursing students and the legal responsibilities they incur?

    a.   They do not need to have professional liability insurance

    b.   They can perform any skill, even if they have not been taught that skill in lab

    c.   They are accountable for any actions they perform

    d.   They practice on the license of their instructor

17. The underlying legal concept that protects the health care professional under the Good Samaritan Act is:

    a.   Informed consent

    b.   Moral consent

    c.   Implied consent

d.   Because it is the ethical thing to do

18.   Which of the following situations might the legal concept of "invasion of privacy" be most likely to exist?

a.   Notification of the police of Mr. Jones' gunshot wound

b.   Discussing Mrs. Green's surgery in the hospital cafeteria

c.   Calling the police concerning an obvious child abuse

d.   Notification of the public health department concerning Mr. Smith's diagnosis of gonorrhea

19   Which of the following situations might a nurse be charged with negligence?

a.   Slapping a patient across the face for using foul language

b.   Not putting the side rails up on a bed of a confused patient

c.   Using restraints on a patient without a doctor's order

d.   Telling the local newspaper of a patient's diagnosis

20.   A nurse is accused of professional negligence. In determining if she is guilty or not, a jury would compare him or her to which of the following standards?

a.   What a physician would have done in the same situation

b.   What a well educated lay person would have done in the same situation

c.   What a reasonable and prudent nurse would have done in the same situation

d.   What a lawyer would have done in the same situation

21. Professional negligence is synonymous with:

    a.   Crime

    b.   Consent

    c.   Misdemeanor

    d.   Malpractice

22. Ms. Jones, RN, is the night charge nurse on your unit. She has come to work this night obviously drunk. As a professional nurse your ethical obligation would be to:

    a.   Ignore her condition out of professional etiquette

    b.   Have a second person validate your observation

    c.   Give her several cups of strong coffee to sober her up

    d.   Have her "sleep it off" in an empty room and cover for her

Answers

1-d	7-d	13-c	19-b
2-c	8-d	14-d	20-c
3-a	9-a	15-d	21-d
4-d	10-c	16-c	22-b
5-b	11-b	17-c	
6-c	12-b	18-b	

CASE STUDY - MAKING ASSIGNMENTS

Maggie C, RN and head nurse of a busy neurological intensive care unit, was reviewing the weekend staffing for the unit on a Friday afternoon. As usual, the unit's nine beds were full with patients in various levels of recovery from brain surgery or head injuries. The staffing on the weekend was "short," with only enough staff to safely care for eight patients. After a great deal of time reworking the schedule, calling nurses on the phone, and trading of days off, she finally managed to arrange sufficient coverage for the unit.

As Maggie was closing her office for the weekend, Dr. West, a neurosurgeon, approached her and related the following situation. Mrs. P, a 63 year old patient with a brain tumor, had been scheduled for surgery three days earlier. She had a very rare blood type that was difficult to match, so the surgery was delayed. Although a few days wait would not likely worsen her condition drastically, she had become very anxious when informed about the delay in surgery. The blood bank had just obtained the necessary units for the surgery and had informed Dr. West that he could now operate on Mrs. P. Dr. West was wondering if the neuro unit would be able to safely care for Mrs. P over the weekend.

This unit was the only unit in the hospital equipped to monitor brain surgery and provide appropriate nursing care for this type of patient. The neuro step-down unit was also full, so it would be difficult getting a bed to transfer one of the neuro units patients into to "make" a bed for Mrs. P. Mrs. P would most likely require one-to-one care for 18 to 24 hours after surgery.

Should Maggie tell Dr. West that he can go ahead with the surgery and she will make the adjustments to provide care for this patient? What ethical obligations does Maggie have to the patient? How about her obligations to Dr. West and the hospital?

(Aiken, TD: <u>Legal, Ethical, and Political Issues In Nursing</u> FA Davis, Philadelphia 1995.)

Additional Critical Thinking Exercises

1. Analyze informed consent as a legal concept and an ethical concept. What are the differences? What are the implications for nurses?

2. Analyze the above three case studies (or any of the case studies in this handbook). What are the legal facts of the case? How might the nurse have prevented a law suit? What is a possible defense the nurse might use?

3. Your mother has just returned from a local hospital where she had an extended stay. She complains of low quality care and has several documented instances where errors were made in nursing and medical care. She wants to sue the hospital, physicians, and nurses, but wants your advice first as a nursing student. What type of advice would you give her? What are your professional, legal, and ethical responsibilities in this situation? Are there any alternatives for a law suit?

4. A nursing colleague working on your unit states: "I've been a nurse for 12 years, have never had malpractice insurance, and have never been sued!" What would be an appropriate response for this statement? Is malpractice insurance necessary?

5. Have the students make a list of incidents they have observed while in their clinical practice that have the potential to become malpractice suits. Discuss ways these incidents might have been changed to lower the potential for a suit.

Chapter 14: Issues in Providing Care

In Chapter 14, the student is acquainted with several of the important issues that affect health care today. A discussion of care delivery models focuses the student's attention on the different structures used in modern health care. The use of computers in health care is discussed. Nursing research is presented as a tool that nurses must be able to use to maximize their ability to make decisions, and improve the quality of care. Legal and ethical obligations in dealing with the chemically impaired nurse are related to the idea of professionalism. The concept of professionalism is further extended to the nurses need to maintain competency in nursing over an extended period of practice. The importance of the image of nursing and how nurses can improve that image is presented. The chapter concludes with a discussion of the future of nursing and how nurses can prepare for it and participate in it.

Teaching Points

1. Present and discuss the different care delivery models used in hospitals and other health care facilities today. Analyze their advantages and disadvantages for nurses.
2. Describe the important functions that computers do and can perform in the delivery of health care. What are the limitations?
3. Discuss the concept of nursing research, and present the different types of research. Identify the students role in research, both as a student and a practicing nurse.
4. List the characteristics that identify the chemically impaired nurse. Discuss the nurse's legal and ethical responsibilities when working with a chemically impaired nurse.

5. Explain why maintaining competency in nursing is important. Distinguish between mandatory and voluntary continuing education and its implications for the profession of nursing.

6. Trace the historical origins for images of nurses. Analyze how these relate to current images of nurses and discuss ways in which nurses can improve their image.

7. Discuss the future of health care and how it influences nursing. How can nurses best prepare for the future?

Questions

1. A type of care delivery model that is task-oriented in that each person performs a specific job to meet a particular need of the unit is called:
    a. Modular nursing
    b. Team nursing
    c. Primary care nursing
    d. Functional nursing

2. A type of care delivery model that focuses on the whole person and gives the nurse responsibility for all of the client's nursing needs is called:
    a. Modular nursing
    b. Team nursing
    c. Primary care nursing
    d. Functional nursing

3. A type of care delivery model that is base on a decentralized organizational system that emphasizes close interdisciplinary collaboration is called:

   a. Modular nursing

   b. Team nursing

   c. Primary care nursing

   d. Functional nursing

4. A type of care delivery model that takes a unified approach to client care involving different levels of care providers working together to achieve client health care goals is called:

   a. Modular nursing

   b. Team nursing

   c. Primary care nursing

   d. Functional nursing

5. Cross-trained personnel are an integral part of which of the following care delivery models?

   a. Team nursing

   b. Modular nursing

   c. Primary care nursing

   d. Functional nursing

6. The primary advantage of the case method of care delivery is:

   a. It is inexpensive and cost effective.

   b. It allows several health care providers trained at different levels to provide care at the same time.

   c. It gives nurses a high degree of autonomy and responsibility.

d.   It allows nurses with minimal education to provide high quality care for all clients.

7.   Which two types of care delivery models are usually used in managed care?
   a.   Functional and team nursing
   b.   Case management and functional nursing
   c.   Modular nursing and primary care nursing
   d.   Case management and primary care nursing

8.   In which of the following health care areas has the use of computers improved the efficiency of care?
   a.   Documentation
   b.   Interdepartmental communication
   c.   Medication administration
   d.   All of the above

9.   The primary concern that health care providers have in the use of computers in client care is:
   a.   The ability to maintain privacy and confidentiality.
   b.   The training and knowledge required by nurses to use the system effectively.
   c.   The ability to provide quality care when the computers malfunction.
   d.   The legal implications of having a computerized record of every aspect of client care.

10. A community health nurse who works with unwed teenage mothers is attempting to determine what common health care practices are used by this group that may affect the health of the fetus. She interviews all the clients she comes in contact with and writes up a report. This would be an example of:

    a.   Quantitative research

    b.   Correlational research

    c.   Qualitative research

    d.   Scientific research

11. Research in health care and nursing is important because:

    a.   It allows nurses to obtain large grants to supplement their low wages.

    b.   It is a way for nurses to improve the quality of client care.

    c.   Its use will impress physicians and improve the image of nursing.

    d.   All of the above.

12. A nurse working the 11 to 7 shift suspects that a coworker has a drug addiction problem. Which of the following symptoms might lead him to this conclusion?

    a.   High quality care and excessive concentration in charting

    b.   Volunteering to give pain medications and refusal of difficult assignments

    c.   Completing assignments and finishing the shift early so that they can go home

    d.   Consistently happy mood and over attention to personal hygiene

13. The primary method of quantifying and recognizing the nurse's attendance, and participation in continuing education programs is:

   a. Granting of academic credit

   b. Awarding of certificates suitable for framing.

   c. Awarding continuing education units

   d. All of the above

14. Which of the following is the most important way that nurses can improve the image of nursing?

   a. Write letters to the television networks and protest programs that portray a negative image for nurses.

   b. Join and support the activities of the professional organizations.

   c. Write to legislators to advocate bills that support professional nursing and nursing education.

   d. Practice nursing with the highest level of professionalism possible.

15. Which of the following aspects of nursing makes it unique in the health care system of today and tomorrow?

   a. Nurses must maintain a high degree of technologic competence in the care of acutely ill clients.

   b. Nursing is primarily a female profession organized and managed by highly educated nurses.

   c. Nursing is the only health care profession that has and can adapt to the many changes in the health care system.

   d. One of the major requirements for nurses is to be able to recognize, and respond to the human response of a client to health care problems.

Answers

1-d	6-c	11-b
2-c	7-d	12-b
3-a	8-d	13-c
4-b	9-a	14-d
5-b	10-c	15-d

CASE STUDY - OVERRIDING AUTONOMY

Mr. Ralph B, a 28 year old factory worker received second and third degree burns over 30 percent of his body when some chemicals he was working with ignited. He survived the initial trauma of these burn injuries and is beginning the long and painful treatment process of debridement, grafting, and rehabilitation. The primary mode of treatment involves twice-a-day whirlpool baths to promote the removal of the dead burned tissue and to promote regeneration of new skin and tissues. For the past two days, even with pretreatment injections of morphine, Ralph has screamed in agony for the whole time he was in the whirlpool bath as well as the post bath dressing procedures. While distressing to the nurses, they are accustomed to the screams of clients, and recognize the need for the baths as a key part of the recovery process.

Upon return to his room after one particularly demonstrative treatment session, Ralph asks the head nurse of the unit to stop taking him for whirlpool treatments. He is lucid, oriented and alert when he makes the request, and makes it clear to the nurse that he understands that refusing the treatments may lead to contractures, poor burn healing, graft rejection, possible infections, and even death. He feels that the agony produced by the treatments far outweigh the benefits he may experience in the future.

The head nurse calls a team conference to discuss the request and discovers that Ralph has been requesting that the whirlpool baths be stopped for over a week. The psychiatrist who is assigned to the burn unit had talked with Ralph several times and feels that he is competent to make decisions about his care. The physician in charge of the case had dealt with clients like Ralph before and feels that the treatments should be continued no matter what the client wants. Nurses are generally considered client advocates. Should

125

the head nurse support the client's decision, or should she support the physician? Are there any alternative solutions for this dilemma?

CASE STUDY - IS AVOIDING THE TRUTH THE SAME AS LYING?

Emma G, 62 years-old, has been a type I diabetic since age 13. Over the years, she had developed many of the long-term complications of diabetes melitis, including a significant loss of vision, poor renal function, high blood pressure, coronary artery disease, and peripheral circulatory problems. A few months ago, she had her right foot and lower leg amputated because of an infection. She was very depressed after this surgery and it took her over a month to recover from her feelings of hopelessness. She still experiences bouts of depression.

She is currently hospitalized with a urinary tract infection and with cyanosis and a draining lesion of her left great toe. The toe is cultured and when the results come back positive for *clostridium*, a common cause for gangrene, she is placed on contact isolation.

Mrs. G is concerned about her condition, and when she asks the nurse why she is in isolation, the nurse tells her that it is because of a urinary tract infection. The nurse felt that it was better to avoid telling the client about the infected toe because of the severe depression she experienced after her amputation of the other leg reasoning that fear of losing her other leg would only increase her stress and may worsen her cardiac status. Both infections were treated with antibiotics, but while the urinary tract infection improved, her whole foot eventually became gangrenous and had to be amputated.

Mrs. G became very angry when she finally learned the truth about her foot, and accused the nurses of lying to her. Did the nurses really lie to Mrs. G? What might have been a better course of action by the nurses in this situation?

Additional Critical Thinking Exercises

1. Have the student select a client they have cared for in the clinical. Based on the clients needs, have the students find a research article that investigates an aspect of the client's condition, and identify methods for incorporating research into client care.

2. List characteristics of leadership which you possess. Which is most important to you? What aspects of your management skills would you like to improve?

3. Prepare a lecture for class. The topic: "How the concept of accountability influences the profession of nursing."

4. Identify the type of care delivery model used in the hospital where the student has clinical practice. What are the advantages or disadvantages of this model for this facility? Are there any alternative models that would work as well or better? Why aren't these models being used?

5. As a class project, have the students make a list of how they feel about computers. Analyze the list with them, discussing the origin of the feeling, and what measures can be used to change that feeling.

6. Have the students contact the state nursing board to find out if their state requires mandatory continuing education. Divide the class into two groups. Have one group take the position that mandatory continuing education is needed and the other groups support voluntary continuing education.

7. Have the students prepare an outline for a fictitious television program that presents a positive image for nurses. What type of plots could be used? What would the setting be? What should be avoided?

Historical Perspectives

The fourteen short sections distributed throughout the book that comprise the *historical perspectives* of the book give an overview of some of the important historical developments in the health care and nursing. They are organized around three common threads, the belief of the cause of disease, the value placed on human life, and the role of women in society.

Many of the problems and difficulties found in the health care system today, in general, and in the profession of nursing, in particular, have their roots in history. A knowledge of these historical roots help the student to understand the profession of nursing, and may suggest solutions to problems that seem unsolvable.

Teaching Points

1. Discuss the importance of history in understanding the current state of health care and nursing.
2. Analyze each *Historical Perspective*, and identify each of the three historical threads that are present.
3. Relate the *Historical Perspective* to some aspect of current health care or nursing practice.

Questions

1. The early Christian era brought which of these important changes in health care?
    a. The development of aqueducts and sewage systems
    b. A belief in the sanctity of life
    c. A deep understanding of the anatomy of the human body

d.   The shift of care from the home to large hospitals

2.   One development during the middle ages that made a significant improvement in health care included:
a.   A rapid growth in medical knowledge
b.   Establishment of large central hospitals
c.   Growth of religious orders to care for the sick
d.   A shift to care for the ill by females

3.   The title "father of modern medicine" is usually attributed to:
a.   William Harvey
b.   Hippocrates
c.   Cyrus the Great
d.   Emperor Darius

4.   Which of the following are the dates of Florence Nightingale birth and death?
a.   March 3, 1578 to June 10, 1657
b.   January 9, 1715 to September 30, 1785
c.   May 12, 1820 to August 13, 1910
d.   April 15, 1932 to December 10, 1957

5.   A key to the success of Nightingale's school of nursing was:
a.   It was not under control of the hospital
b.   Large amounts of private funds to pay well qualified teachers
c.   Use of the Watson Model for nursing
d.   The primary goal of service to the hospital rather than education

6.   A major goal of Lavinia Dock during her life time was to:

    a.   Establish a new nursing organization

    b.   Publish a nursing journal

    c.   Obtain the right to vote for women

    d.   Improve the education for nurses

7.   Ms. Lillian D. Wald believed strongly that nurses need to:

    a.   Spend more time in clinical preparation and less time in the class room.

    b.   Fight political corruption to procure the types of legislation needed to improve social conditions.

    c.   Conduct more research into the conditions of hospital patients.

    d.   Stand up to medical doctors who were arrogant and obnoxious.

8.   A significant problem in nursing education during the 1920s and 1930s was:

    a.   Too many college based schools of nursing

    b.   A lack of qualified nursing instructors

    c.   Too many nursing students from the lower and middle class

    d.   Not enough demand for educated nurses

9.   A negative effect that World War II had on health care in the United States was:

    a.   A rapid increase in medical knowledge

    b.   Expanded health care services

    c.   Increase use of LPN's and aids to substitute for lower numbered of RNs

    d.   Increases in pay for nurses

10.   Which of the following are the statements concerning the effects of increasing populations on health care?

    a.   The economically depressed populations have more health care needs.

    b.   Larger populations often lead to large numbers of poor, uneducated and under-nourished people.

    c.   Large groups of economically depressed tend to converge in cities.

    d.   All of the above.

Answers

1-b	6-c
2-c	7-b
3-a	8-b
4-c	9-c
5-a	10-d

CASE STUDY

After her initial 6 week orientation period, Patty N a new graduate RN, was beginning her first job on the 11 to 7 shift in a busy surgical unit of a city hospital. Patty enjoyed the busy pace of the unit, the development of new skills in the care of complicated postoperative patients, and the spirit of cooperation and camaraderie with the other nurses on the shift. She particularly liked to see the patients recover and resume a normal life.

Because of the nature of the surgical unit and the fact that most of the patients were in pain to some degree, large quantities of narcotics and other pain medications were used. Occasionally the narcotic count was "off" at the end of the shift, but the nurses were usually able to track down who forgot to "sign-out" a medication. After several weeks of working on the unit, Patty began to notice that the narcotic count was always wrong when Vickie L, an older RN who had worked on the unit for five years, was working. Patty also noticed that Vickie signed out pain medications for her patients at the minimal intervals ordered all through the shift, even if the patient had not received any medication for the previous 24 hours.

Patty asked one of the other nurses about Vickie. Patty was told by the nurse that Vickie was an excellent nurse, a hard worker, and would be virtually impossible to replace if she were to leave or be fired. It was also related to Patty that she was the newcomer to the unit and that she really should not "make waves." If Patty really wanted to help, she was informed that she could "cover" for Vickie, as the other nurses did, when she was "sick," which was often.

After observing Vickie more closely, Patty recognized the symptoms of drug abuse that she had been taught in school, including moody and erratic behavior, frequent absences because of "illness," forgetting to give scheduled medications on time, and frequent and prolonged "bathroom" breaks throughout the shift. Patty felt that Vickie's behavior and problem were dangerous to the patients she was caring for.

What should Patty do? What are the key elements in this ethical dilemma? What does the Code of Ethics for Nurses say about incompetent practitioners? Are there any legal and/or ethical obligations that apply to Patty's actions?

(Aiken, TD: Legal, Ethical, and Political Issues In Nursing FA Davis, Philadelphia 1995.)

Critical Thinking Exercises

1. Delineate and discuss those factors found in history that encourage and support the evolution of nursing as a profession.

2. Apply the convictions of the early nursing leaders to the nursing profession as it is practiced today. Identify the similarities and the differences.

3. Wars have always had a profound effect on health care and nursing. Discuss the common elements found in the Crusades, Revolutionary War, Civil War, World War I, and World War II that influence the health care and nursing practice of today.

4. What elements of primitive and ancient health care are important to health care today. Are any of these elements a part of current practices?

5. Throughout history, religion has often had a profound effect on health care practices. Identify key religious practices that influenced health care in the past. Are there any situations today where religion has an effect on health care?

6. Why are most nurses women in today's health care system? What are the historical origins of this fact?